ATLAS OF LAPAROSCOPIC UROLOGIC SURGERY

ATLAS OF LAPAROSCOPIC UROLOGIC SURGERY

Edited by

Jan Roigas
Klinik und Poliklinik für Urologie
Berlin
Germany

Serder Deger
Klinik und Poliklinik für Urologie
Charité – Universitätsmedizin Berlin
Berlin
Germany

Stefan A Loening
Klinik und Poliklinik für Urologie
Charité – Universitätsmedizin Berlin
Berlin
Germany

Andreas H Wille
Department of Urology
University Hospital Charité
Humboldt-University Berlin
Berlin
Germany

CRC Press
Taylor & Francis Group
Boca Raton London New York

CRC Press is an imprint of the
Taylor & Francis Group, an **informa** business

First published 2009 by Informa Healthcare USA, Inc.

Published 2021 by CRC Press
Taylor & Francis Group
6000 Broken Sound Parkway NW, Suite 300
Boca Raton, FL 33487-2742

ISBN 13: 978-1-8418-4541-8 (hbk)

Visit the Taylor & Francis Web site at
http://www.taylorandfrancis.com

and the CRC Press Web site at
http://www.crcpress.com

Contents

Contributors

Chr Assenmacher
Department of Urology
Onze-Lieve-Vrouw Hospital
Aalst
Belgium

Alexander Bachmann
Department of Urology
University Hospital Basel
Basel
Switzerland

Renaud Bollens
Department of Urology
Onze-Lieve-Vrouw Hospital
Aalst
Belgium

Serdar Deger
Klinik und Poliklinik für Urologie
Charité - Universitätsmedizin Berlin
Berlin
Germany

Peter Dekuyper
Department of Urology
Onze-Lieve-Vrouw Hospital
Aalst
Belgium

Anja Dietel
Department of Urology
University of Leipzig
Leipzig
Germany

Minh Do
Department of Urology
University of Leipzig
Leipzig
Germany

M Fillet
Department of Urology
Onze-Lieve-Vrouw Hospital
Aalst
Belgium

Franco Gaboardi
Department of Urologic Surgery
Luigi Sacco University Medical Center
Milan
Italy

Stefano Galli
Department of Urologic Surgery
Luigi Sacco University Medical Center
Milan
Italy

Markus Giessing
Department of Urology
Charité University Hospital
Berlin
Germany

Joannes Goumas
Department of Urologic Surgery
Luigi Sacco University Medical Center
Milan
Italy

Andrea Gregori
Department of Urologic Surgery
Luigi Sacco University Medical Center
Milan
Italy

Evangelos N Liatsikos
Department of Urology
University of Leipzig
Leipzig
Germany

P Martens
Department of Urology
Onze-Lieve-Vrouw Hospital
Aalst
Belgium

Alan McNeill
Department of Urology
University of Leipzig
Leipzig
Germany

Alexander Mottrie
Department of Urology
Onze-Lieve-Vrouw Hospital
Aalst
Belgium

H Nicholas
Department of Urology
Onze-Lieve-Vrouw Hospital
Aalst
Belgium

Robert Rabenalt
Department of Urology
University of Leipzig
Leipzig
Germany

Jan Roigas
Klinik and Poliklinik für Urologie
Berlin
Germany

Robin Ruszat
Department of Urology
University Hospital Basel
Basel
Switzerland

Jens-Uwe Stolzenburg
Department of Urology
University of Leipzig
Leipzig
Germany

Roland Van Velthoven
Department of Urology
Onze-Lieve-Vrouw Hospital
Aalst
Belgium

Andreas H Wille
Department of Urology
University Hospital Charité
Humboldt-University Berlin
Berlin
Germany

Mario Zacharias
Department of Urology
University Clinic Eppendorf
Hamburg
Germany

Preface

In the last decade, laparoscopy has undergone a revolutionary develoment in urologic surgery. Starting from initial case reports and small patient series of experienced centers, a variety of complex laparoscopic urologic procedures, like tumor nephrectomy, donor nephrectomy, and radical prostatectomy, have been declared as a second standard beside the corresponding open procedures. Also, radical cystectomy and urinary diversion, the most challenging urooncological procedure, has been the focus of the laparoscopic approach.

Laparoscopic urologic surgery, combined with fast-track surgical approaches, seems to improve patients' perioperative quality of life. Almost all oncological and reconstructive operations are now in the repertoire of the laparoscopic approach.

The excellent view due to the magnification allows for delicate anatomic preparation, resulting in less tissue trauma and minimal blood loss. Trans- or extraperitoneal and even robotic-assisted surgical approaches have been developed and are currently undergoing further clinical distribution.

All these matters are well known by urologists, who were always seeking minimally invasive procedures, such as transurethral resection of prostatic hyperplasia and the bladder cancers, extracorporeal shock wave lithotripsy, and percutaneous and endoscopic techniques.

Rapid changes in a short time period and the establishment of different techniques brought the problem of teaching this new tool in the urologic community. The teaching capability of laparoscopic surgery is an important, if not the most important, aspect for the further distribution and acceptance of laparoscopy in urology.

Our *Atlas of Laparoscopic Urologic Surgery* aims to present established procedures not only to beginners but also to urologists who have already made their first steps in this field and are looking to expand. We have tried to describe established procedures in a step by step fashion using illustrations and intraoperative photos without presenting a heavy textbook. The trainee can easily find his path through illustrations with instructions, tips, and tricks of the procedure, described by experienced laparoscopic surgeons.

We hope our atlas will help to further propagate laparoscopic techniques in the urologic community.

Stefan Leoning
Jan Roigas

Part I Laparoscopic Surgery of the Kidney

CHAPTER I

Retroperitoneal access

Alexander Bachmann and Robin Ruszat

INTRODUCTION

Since its introduction in 1990 by Clayman et al.[1] laparoscopic nephrectomy is being increasingly performed at numerous institutions worldwide. When removal of kidney is indicated for a benign pathological condition laparoscopic nephrectomy has largely superseded the traditional open approach. One of the major advantages of the retroperitoneoscopic approach is the quick access to the vessels, without any interference of bowel, liver, spleen, or adhesions. The need to mobilize the ascending or descending colon is obviated. The most frequent arguments against the retroperitoneoscopic approach are the difficulty in establishing the topography, the smaller working space, and the steeper learning curve compared with the transperitoneal approach.

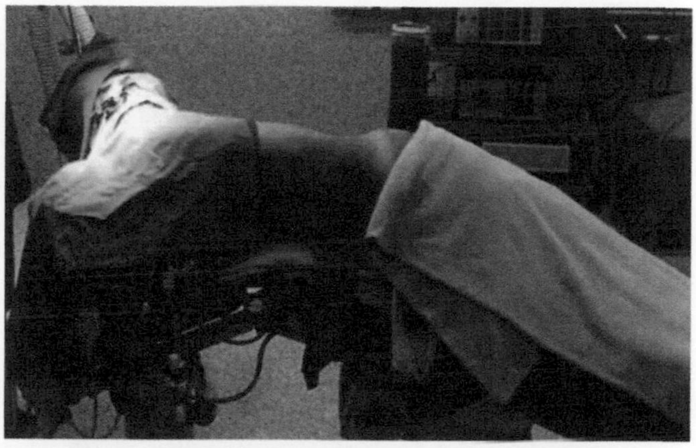

Figure 1.1 The patient is positioned in the standard full-flank position with the kidney rest elevated and the operative table flexed. This maximizes the space between the iliac crest and the 12th rib.

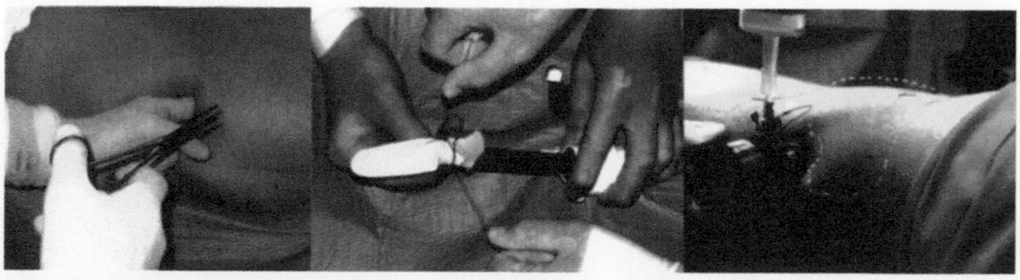

Figure 1.2 At the tip of the 12th rib a skin incision is made and the initial retroperitoneal space is created bluntly by index finger dissection. A straight Kocher's clamp is ideal for gentle and controlled perforation of the deep fascia and the quadratus lumborum ligament instead of using a scissor or scalpel, because the index finger can guide the instrument safely. Afterwards the dissection balloon is inserted. This self-made dissection balloon is an efficient tool for all kinds of extraperitoneal sugery. At the tip of the trocar sheet two separated surgical glove fingers, that are placed one inside the other, are fixed with twine. Finally 800–1000 ml (cold) sterile saline solution is injected. The anterior hump (dotted line) is visible as a sign of correct extraperitoneal space dissection. If no hump is visible, the balloon is not placed correctly (probably intraperitoneal). After removal of the balloon dissector, a pneumoperitoneum is established with an intra-abdominal pressure of 12–15 mmHg.

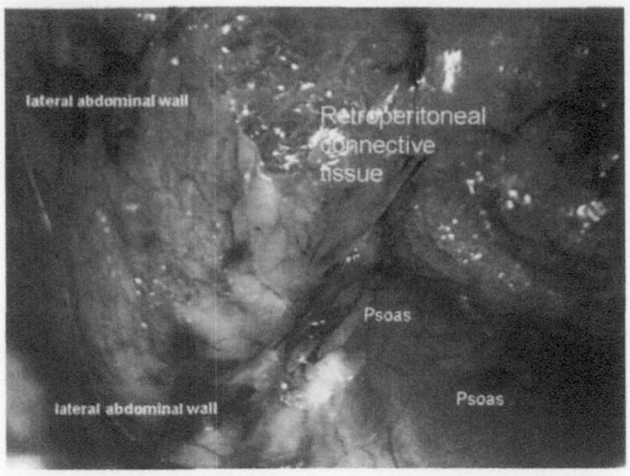

Figure 1.3 Initial extraperitoneal endoscopic (syn: retroperitoneoscopic) appearance after blunt retroperitoneal balloon dissection. The psoas muscle is one of the most important landmarks in retroperitoneal orientation and usually appears horizontally on the video screen. In case of disorientation because of bleeding or excessive perirenal fatty tissue, the surgeon should come back to the psoas muscle to get an anatomic overview.

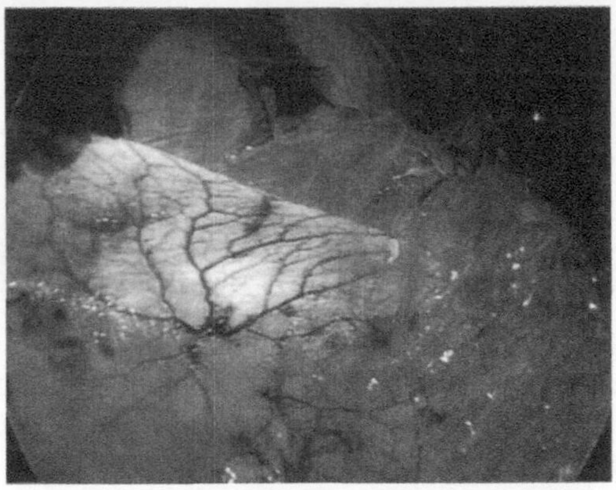

Figure 1.4 By turning the 30° optical system of the laparoscope upwards to the abdominal wall, the peritoneal reflexion is easily identified. The peritoneum is softly dissected medio-ventrally using the tip of the camera. In order to control the position of the camera tip and to prevent injury of the peritoneum it is important that the dissection is controlled by the surgeon's other hand on the outer abdominal wall.

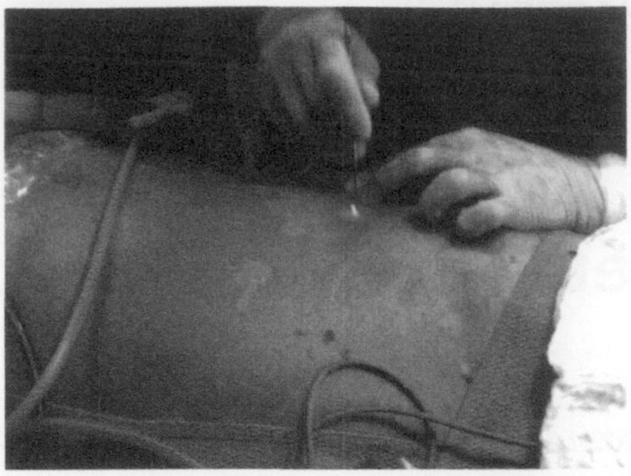

Figure 1.5 After the peritoneal border is dissected medially, via diaphanoscopy the second trocar is localized just a few centimeters above and medial to the superior anterior iliac spine. Usually a 10 or 12 mm trocar is inserted at this position.

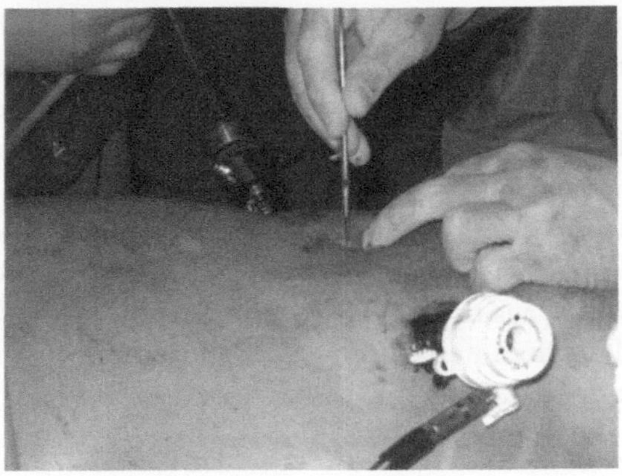

Figure 1.6 The third 5 mm trocar is inserted just in the middle between the two trocars that have already been inserted. Sometime it is advisable to insert the third trocar a little bit more laterally in this connection line, because the working angle is more comfortable. A fourth trocar is optional; however, it is advisable in complex surgery.

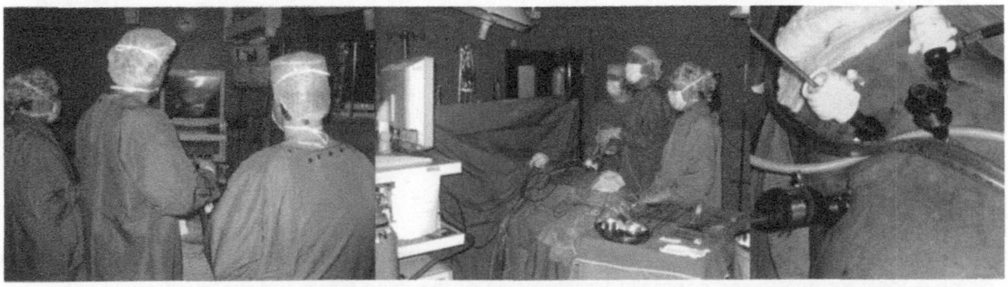

Figure 1.7 The surgeon, the assistant, and the theatre nurse are positioned dorsally to the patient. The video tower is placed in front of the patient. The assistant is holding the camera and serving the optional fourth trocar (blue rubber in the right lateral picture). Finally, four trocars are placed in a classic rhombus position.

REFERENCE

1. Clayman RV, Kavoussi LR, Figenshau RS, Chandhoke PS, Albala DM. Laparoscopic nephroureterectomy: Initial clinical case report. J Laparoendosc Surg 1991; 1: 343–9.

CHAPTER 2

Laparoscopic fenestration of lymphoceles

Markus Giessing

INDICATION

A lymphocele (LCs) is a collection of lymphatic fluid in a cavity that is not lined by epithelium. *They* occur after lymphadenectomy, mostly performed as staging lymphadenectomy in prostatic cancer or in the context of cystectomy and after kidney transplantation. Risk factors for forming LCs are heparin given into the thigh and insufficient intraoperative ligation of lymphatic vessels. The reasons for development of LCs following kidney transplantation remain unclear, as the donor's kidney as well as the recipient's lymphatics may contribute to their formation. In the context of kidney transplantation, rejection episodes and immunosuppression including the mTOR-inhibitor sirolimus are additional risk factors.[1]

About two-thirds of the LCs remain asymptomatic. Clinical symptoms of a LC mostly develop secondary to compression of blood vessels and include edema of the leg, thrombosis, and pulmonary embolism. Obstruction of the transplant ureter with consecutive urinary tract obstruction and reduced graft function may occur. Large LCs can cause abdominal pain. Infection of LCs can develop and is associated with fever and pain.

Studies have shown that transperitoneal fenestration (plus omentoplasty) is the best therapy for uninfected LCs,[2,3] as alternative therapeutic options such as drainage plus instillation[4] or open fenestration keep the patient immobile and hospitalized for longer. Infection and urine collection/urinoma must be excluded to the operation by puncture (creatinine, microbiology/sediment). Infected LCs should be treated by drainage, and urinomas by ureteral stenting, Foley catheter, and possibly a further operation like a new uretero-cysto-neostomy (re-UCN). The only contraindication to laparoscopic LC fenestration – besides infection and urinoma – is an inoperable localization.[5]

PREOPERATIVE SCHEDULE

- CT or MRI for exact localization
- Exclusion of infection/urinoma by puncture (creatinine, Gram stain, culture) by Doppler ultrasound
- Exclusion of a venous thrombosis (liberation of venous bloodstream may cause pulmonary embolism)
- 18:00/20:00 enema
- 20:00 only anticoagulation s.c.
- Suprapubic depilation/cleaning of umbilicus.

INSTRUMENTATION

- Basic laparoscopy set:
  - trocars: $2 \times 10/1 \times 5$ mm
  - laparoscopy coagulation device (bipolar is best)
  - laparoscopy graspers, scissors
  - laparoscopy aspiration needle
  - laparoscopy suction device
  - laparoscopy needle holder
- Suture:
  - for omentoplasty (4×0 Vycril/Lahotny suture)
- Optional:
  - preoperative ureteral stenting.

STEP-BY-STEP OPERATIVE TECHNIQUE

- Single-shot cortisone and antibiotic prophylaxis for protection of the kidney transplant
- Optional: preoperative ureteral stenting
- Three trocar transperitoneal technique
- Sterile bladder catheterization for optional bladder filling intraoperatively.

POSTOPERATIVE SCHEDULE

- Day of operation
  mobilization 4–6 hours after operation
  urinary output control
  yoghurt and tea (time according to anesthesiologist's recommendations)/add infusions
  thrombosis prophylaxis
  pain medication.
- Postoperative day 1
  ultrasound transplant and exclude residual LC
  serum creatinine
  light diet/no further infusion
  complete mobilization
  thrombosis prophylaxis
  pain medication.
- Postoperative day 2
  discharge (when no complications have occurred).

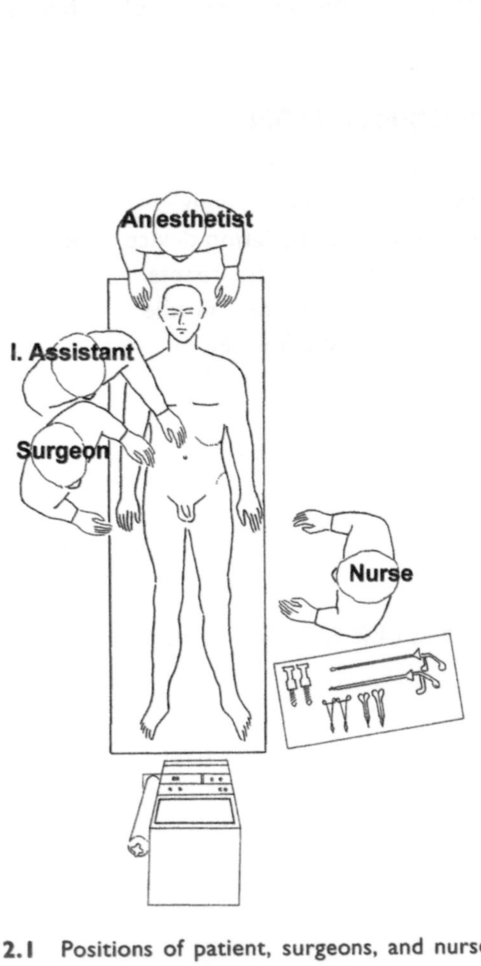

Figure 2.1 Positions of patient, surgeons, and nurse in the operation room: one surgeon/one assistant contralateral to the LC side, and one nurse on the LC side.

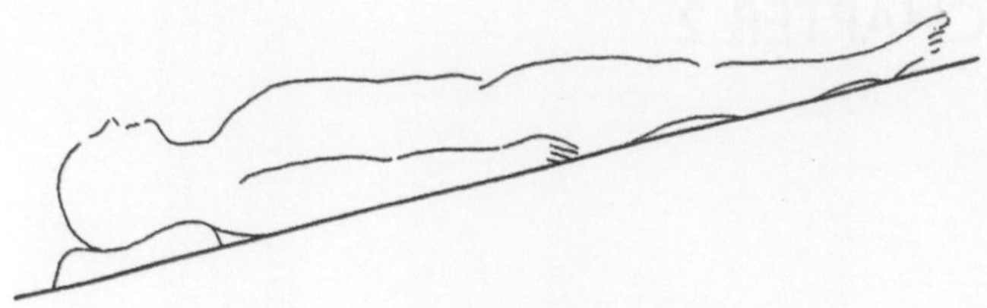

Figure 2.2 Position of the patient on the operation table: positioned on the back, arms extended.

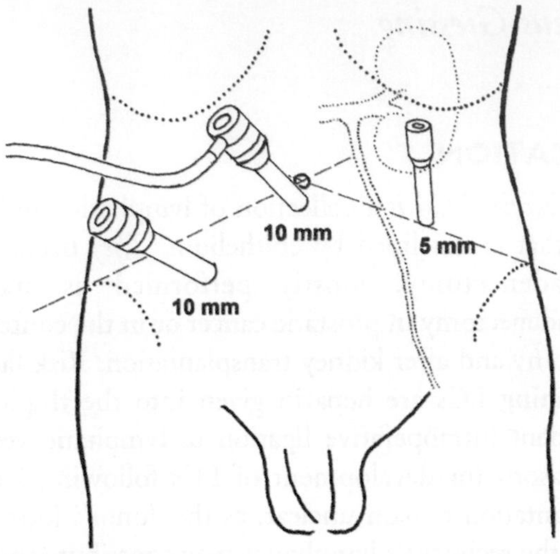

Figure 2.3 Position of the trocars for the operation field: 10 mm optical trocar infra-umbilical; 10 mm trocar contralateral to LC in medio-clavicular line at spina iliaca anterior superior; 5 mm trocar: between optical trocar and LC.

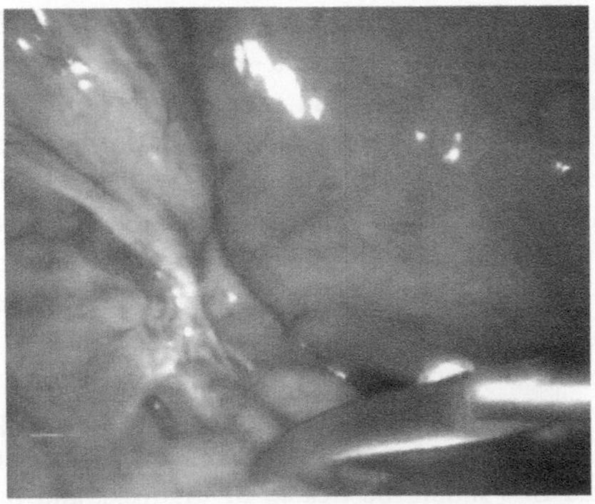

Figure 2.4 Mobilizing adherent tissue. For access to the lymphocele the adherent tissue has to be dissected. For orientation in the situs it may be helpful to fill up the urinary bladder via the inlaying Foley catheter. If a drain is in the lymphocele (after a failed drainage and sclerosing therapy), filling up the LC via the drain may be helpful. Adding a dye (e.g. indigocarmine/methylene blue) to the saline chloride for filling up the bladder or the LC increases the detectability of accidental lesions during the operation. In difficult cases intraoperative ultrasound is recommended.

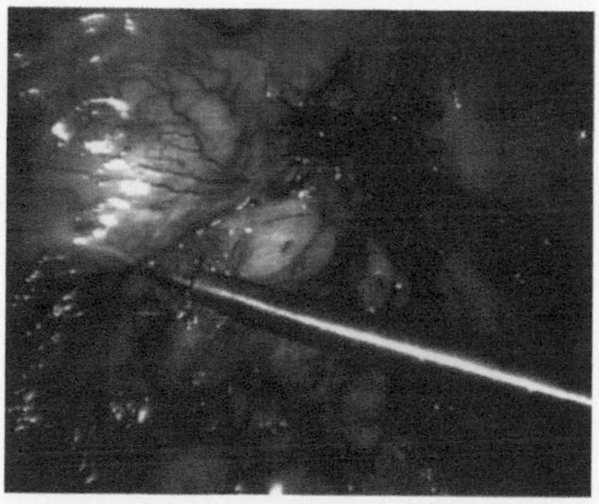

Figure 2.5 Identification of the lymphocele by puncture. To clearly identify the correct structure puncture of the LC is performed. The fluid should be amber-colored and should be sent for microbiological examination in case of postoperative infectious complications. Accidental puncture of the transplant or of the iliac vessels may occur but is rarely followed by complications.

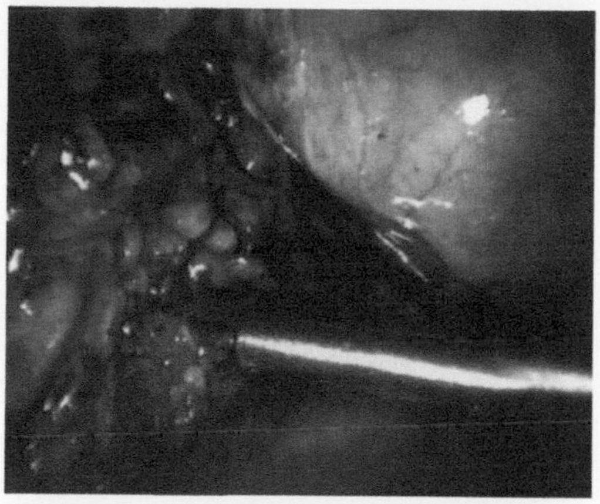

Figure 2.6 Complete dissection of the lymphocele. Once the LC is clearly identified via puncture the adherent tissue is dissected.

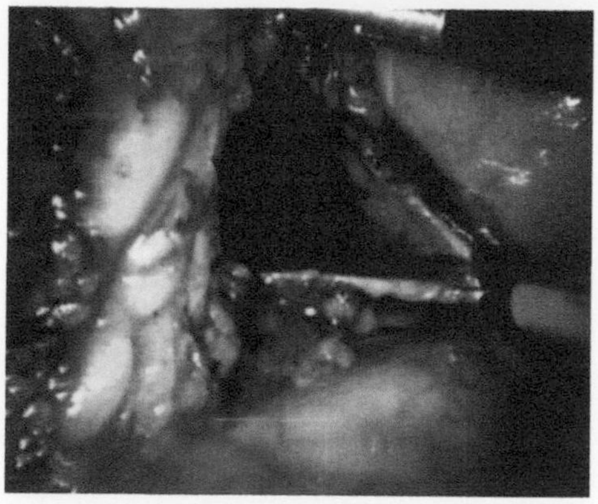

Figure 2.7 Opening of the lymphocele. The complete medial wall of the LC is opened with grasper and scissors. Care must be taken not to injure the vessels or the transplant ureter. Once the complete wall of the LC is identified it is cut off. The camera can now go into the LC and septa can be destroyed. Histology does not necessarily have to be performed except for proof of the action. Coagulation of the complete border of the LC with bipolar forceps is recommended, as this is the region at risk for bleedings.

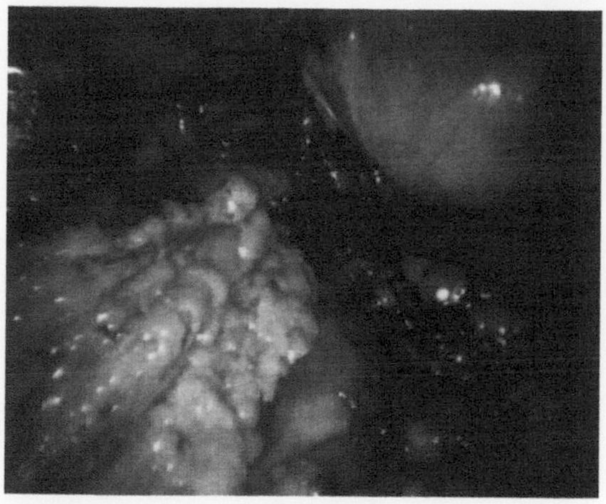

Figure 2.8 Omentoplasty. To reduce the risk of reformation of the LC, omentum is mobilized and fixed in the cavity of the LC. Suture is performed with 4 × 0 Vicryl or Lahotny suture. In case of a very short omentum it can be lengthened by a T-like incision with the GIA stapler. Note that trocars are removed under vision to exclude incisional bleedings, for trocars larger than 10 mm the fascia should be sutured under visual control. Complete desufflation is carried out at the end of the operation to prevent abdominal and shoulder pain. Skin closure can be performed with intracutaneous fast resorbable sutures.

REFERENCES

1. Giessing M, Fischer T, Deger S et al. Increased frequency of lymphoceles under treatment with sirolimus following renal transplantation: a single center experience. Transplant Proc 2002; 34: 1815–16.
2. Fuller TF, Kang SM, Hirose et al. Management of lymphoceles after renal transplantation: laparoscopic versus open drainage. J Urol 2003; 169: 2022–5.
3. Bailey SH, Mone MC, Holman JM et al. Laparoscopic treatment of postrenal transplant lymphoceles. Surg Endosc 2003; 17: 1896–9.
4. Caliendo M, Lee DE, Queiroz R. Sclerotherapy with use of doxycycline after percutaneous drainage of postoperative lymphoceles. J Vasc Interv Radiol 2001; 12: 73–7.
5. Gil IS, Hodge EE, Munch LC et al. Transperitoneal marsupialization of lymphoceles: a comparison of laparoscopic and open techniques. J Urol 1995; 153: 706–11.

CHAPTER 3

Retroperitoneoscopic radical tumor nephrectomy

Alexander Bachmann and Robin Ruszat

INDICATION

Indications for retroperitoneoscopic tumor nephrectomy are organ-confined renal tumors, stage T1-(2). Large tumor size is only a relative contraindication, which depends on the comfort level of the surgeon and the individual characteristics of the tumor. Contraindications include vena caval thrombus, bulky lymphadenopathy, locally invasive tumors, and previous excessive lumbal surgery.

PREOPERATIVE SCHEDULE

The patient reports to the hospital 1 day before surgery and undergoes routine preoperative evaluation including blood analysis, chest X-ray, and electrocardiography. Special bowel preparation is not necessary for retroperitoneoscopy. To prevent thrombosis the patient receives subcutaneous low-molecular-weight heparin on the evening before the operation. One hour preoperatively broad-spectrum antibiotics are administered intravenously. Following general anesthesia and Foley catheter placement, the patient is safely secured to the operating table in a standard full-flank position.

STEP-BY-STEP OPERATIVE TECHNIQUE

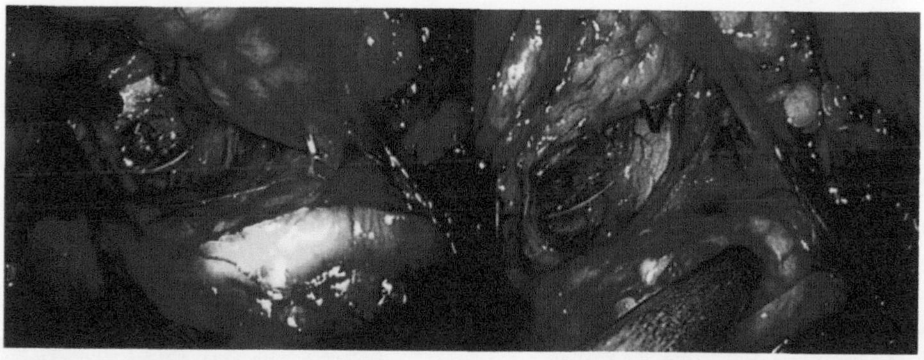

Figure 3.1 After the Gerota's fascia is horizontally incised the renal hilum can be easily identified by renal artery pulsations. Dissection of renal artery and vein is performed using monopolar scissors, bipolar forceps or harmonic scalpels. The covering lymphatic tissue is carefully dissected from the artery. The vein (V) is always identified behind the artery (A), as seen in the right-hand picture. Close to the kidney the ureter (U) is identifiable (left-hand picture, tip of the suction device).

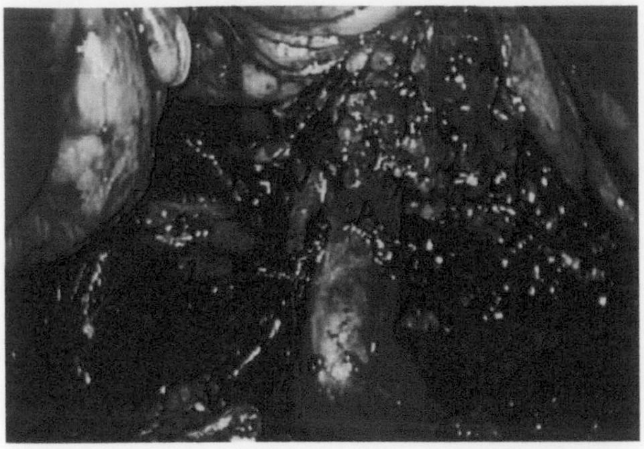

Figure 3.2 First the renal artery (A) is sufficiently freed from lymphatic and fatty tissue and circumferentially mobilized. At this stage, as seen in the picture, the vessels are ready for transection. V, vein.

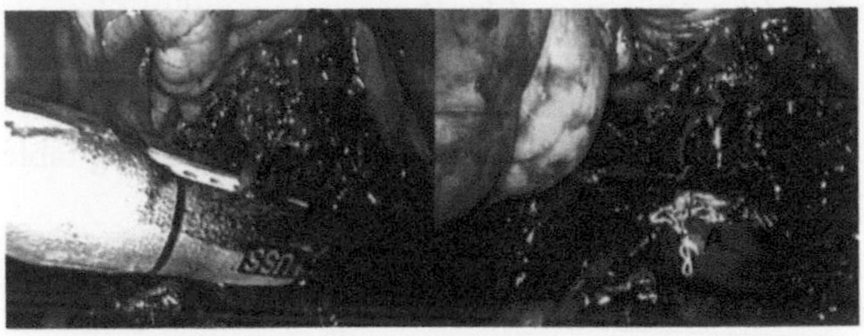

Figure 3.3 Transection of the renal artery (A) and vein (V) can be safely performed using angled or non-angled cutting staplers. Artery and vein are transected separately.

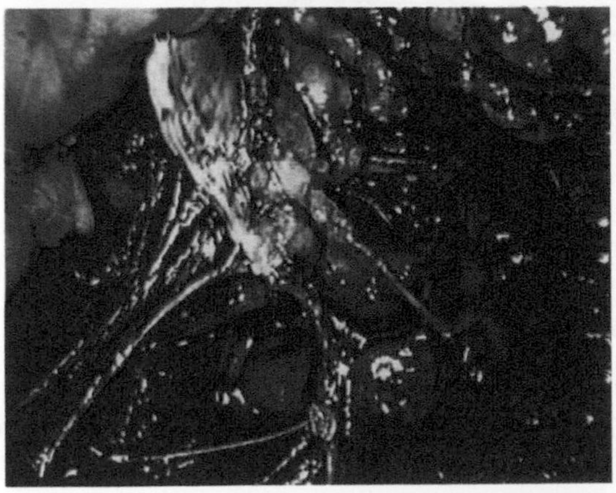

Figure 3.4 Finally both vessels are transected and the entire kidney is lifted medially, because it is still fixed to the peritoneum with its anterior surface. Dissection is next directed towards the craniolateral aspect of the specimen, including if necessary en bloc adrenal gland, which is readily mobilized from the underside of the diaphragm. Inferior phrenic vessels to the adrenal gland are frequently encountered in the avascular tissue in this location and have to be controlled.

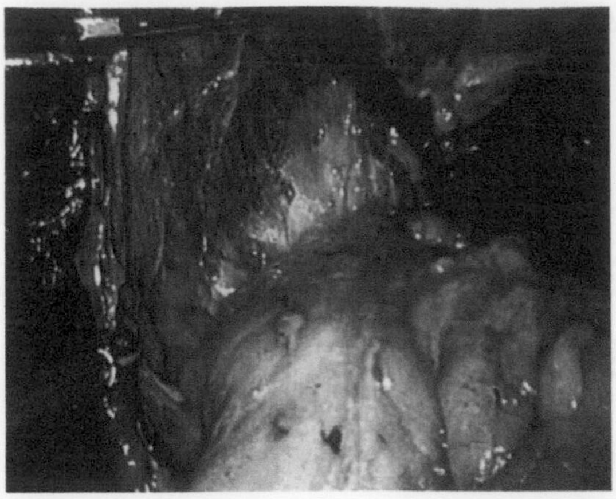

Figure 3.5 The entire dissection is performed outside the Gerota's fascia to ensure the oncological principles of open surgery. After clip occlusion the ureter is divided and the specimen is entrapped in an Endo-catch bag and extracted intact by enlarging the secondary port side appropriately. We do not perform morcellation for any cancer. Hemostasis is confirmed under lowered pneumoretroperitoneum and ports are removed in a routine manner.

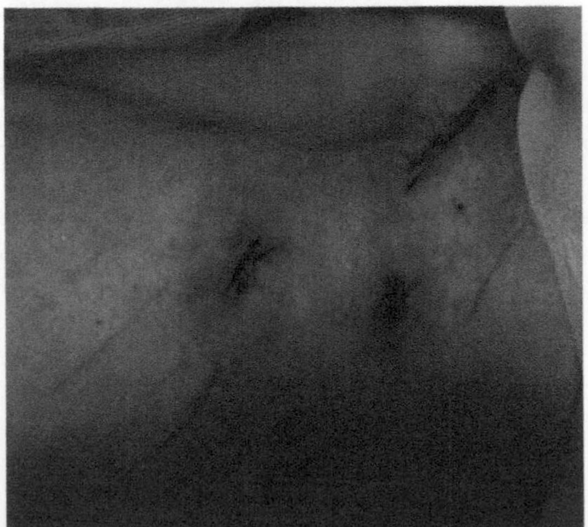

Figure 3.6

CHAPTER 4

Laparoscopic radical tumor nephrectomy – transperitoneal approach

Jan Roigas

INDICATION

The indication for laparoscopic tumor nephrectomy for small renal masses (< 7 cm, category T1) is similar to open surgery and mainly includes centrally localized tumors in which an organ-preserving concept is technically not possible.

Renal masses between 7 and 10 cm can be treated with the laparoscopic approach, but the size of the renal mass often limits access to the renal hilum and the intraoperative handling of the organ. Therefore, indication should be strict and the surgeon should be well experienced with laparoscopic procedures.

Renal masses larger than 10 cm or tumors with preoperatively diagnosed renal or caval vein involvement should not be treated by laparoscopy. Here, experienced centers are currently investigating the feasibility of the laparoscopic approach.

Principally the laparoscopic technique mimics the steps of open surgery with:

- mobilization of the colon
- identification of the ureter
- preparation of the renal hilum
- transection of the renal artery and renal vein
- transection of the ureter
- complete mobilization of the kidney with tumor, fat capsule, adrenal gland, and hiliac lymph nodes
- extraction of the specimen via a muscle-splitting mini incision.

The role of an extended lymph node dissection and the removal of the adrenal gland can be similarly discussed for open and laparoscopic surgery.

PREOPERATIVE SCHEDULE

- Diet: Patients can have normal breakfast in the morning, soup for lunch, and fluid only in the evening.
- Bowel preparation: No specific bowel preparation is necessary. Two rectal enemas are administered in the evening.
- Perioperative antibiotic treatment: Third-generation cephalosporin is used as a single shot during surgery.

INSTRUMENTATION

- 1 trocar (10 mm)
- 1 trocar (5 mm or 10 mm)
- 1 trocar (5 mm)
- 1 trocar (5 mm) optional
- optical system (10 mm, 30°) for first assistant
- scissors for surgeon
- grasper for surgeon.

PATIENT POSITION

Figure 4.1 shows the organization of the patient and the personnel in the operating room. Prior to positioning a transurethral catheter should be placed into the urinary bladder. Then the patient is placed on the non-tumor side in a lateral decubitus position with a 45° angle and a flexed operating table (see Figures 4.2, 4.3, and 4.4). This angle is critical, because a very steep position (> 45°) leads to a dislocation of the kidney with the fat capsule in the direction of the renal hilum, which renders the preparation of these structures more difficult. Before the infra-umbilical incision, the table has to be tilted to the side away from the surgeon. This leads to a

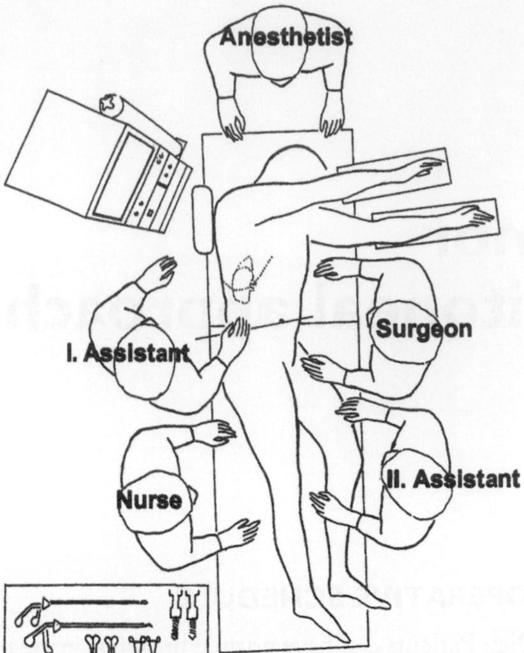

Figure 4.1 Layout of the operating room showing the position of the patient and the personnel.

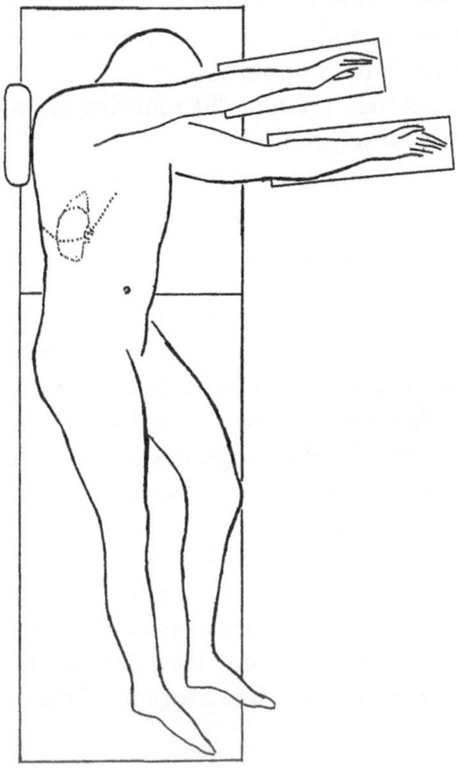

Figure 4.2 The patient is positioned on the healthy side.

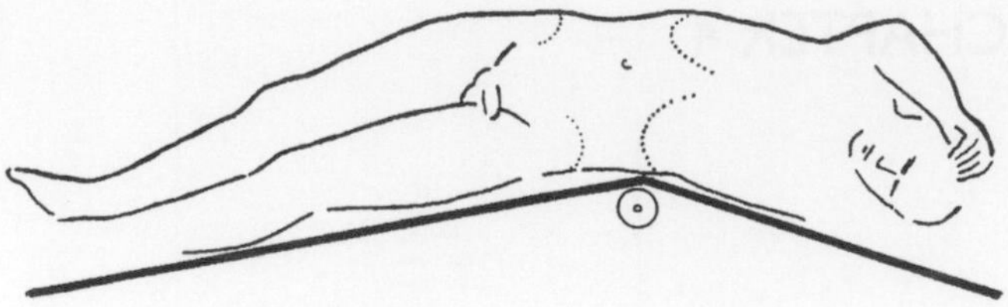

Figure 4.3 The table is flexed.

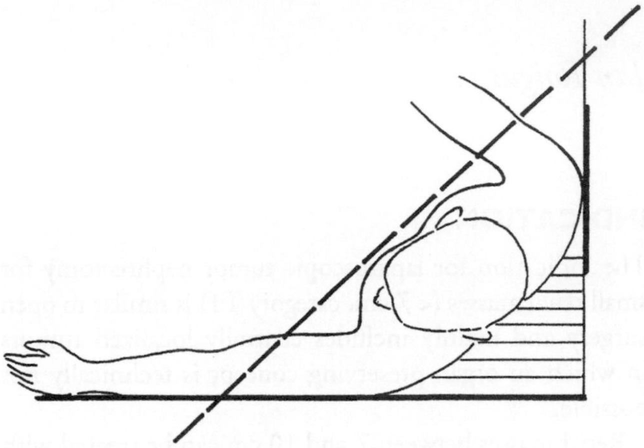

Figure 4.4 The angle should be at about 45°.

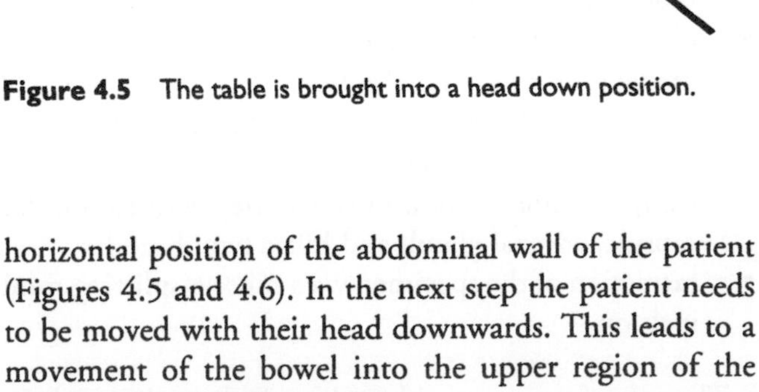

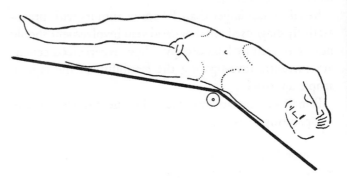

Figure 4.5 The table is brought into a head down position.

horizontal position of the abdominal wall of the patient (Figures 4.5 and 4.6). In the next step the patient needs to be moved with their head downwards. This leads to a movement of the bowel into the upper region of the abdominal cavity (Figure 4.7).

For the surgeon, the patient now appears to lie on his back and the abdominal wall can easily be lifted up (Figures 4.8 and 4.9). In this manner, the infra-umbilical incision can be made and a Veress needle can be placed into the abdominal cavity (Figure 4.10).

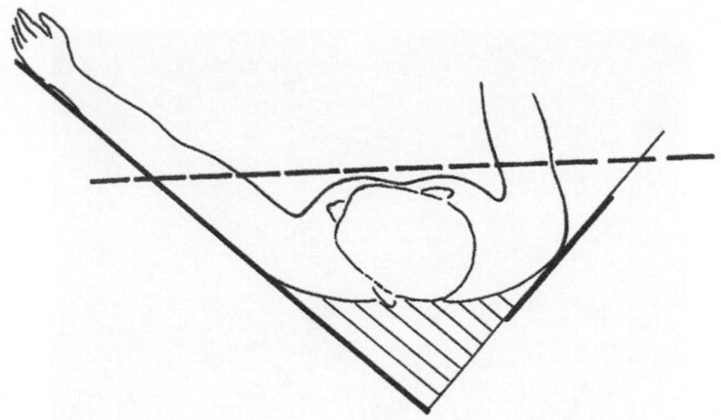

Figure 4.6 The table is turned away from the surgeon.

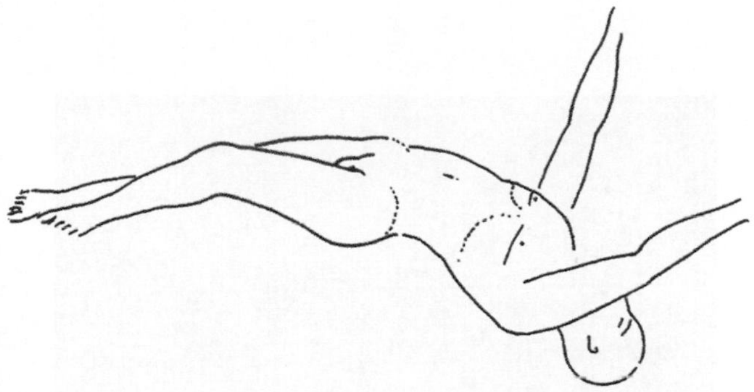

Figure 4.7 The patient is in a position with the abdominal wall up.

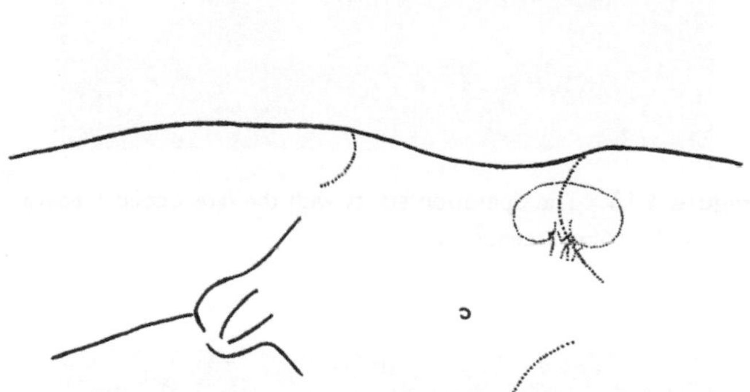

Figure 4.8 For the surgeon, the patient appears to lie on his back.

TROCAR PLACEMENT

A four-trocar technique positioned as shown in Figure 4.11 can be used. The 10 mm optical trocar is placed in the infra-umbilical region, followed by the placement of a 5 mm trocar in the upper medioclavicular line and a 10 or 12 mm trocar for the use of an Endo-GIA in the lower

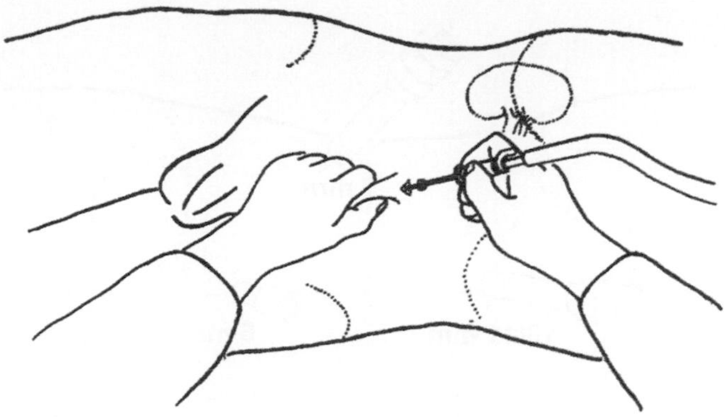

Figure 4.9 The infra-umbilical incision can be made and the Veress needle can be placed.

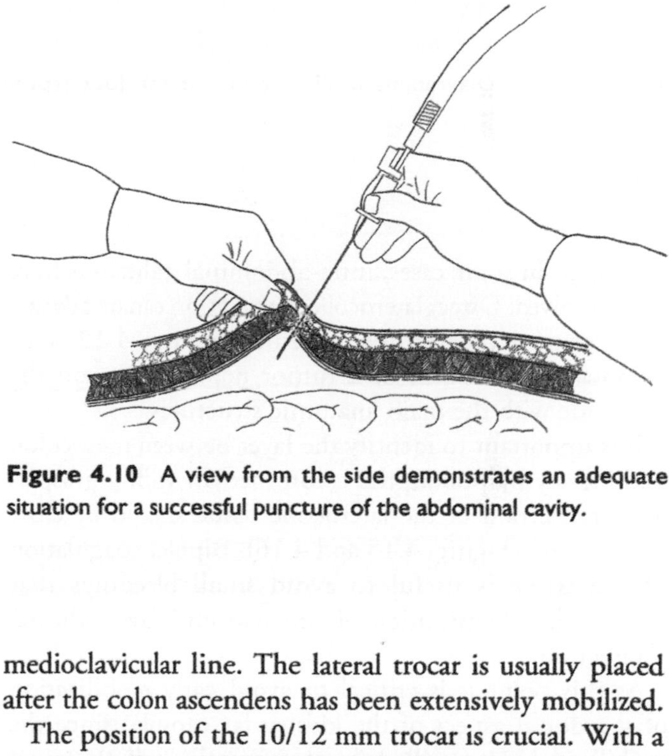

Figure 4.10 A view from the side demonstrates an adequate situation for a successful puncture of the abdominal cavity.

medioclavicular line. The lateral trocar is usually placed after the colon ascendens has been extensively mobilized.

The position of the 10/12 mm trocar is crucial. With a very cranially positioned trocar the formation of an equilateral triangle is not possible and the optic trocar and the 12 mm trocar will hinder each other, especially when the use of the 30° camera angle is required for renal preparation of the hilum. On the other hand, if the trocar is placed very caudally, the preparation of the upper pole of the kindey can be difficult. In addition, at this position access to the renal vein for transection with the Endo-GIA can be difficult.

OPERATIVE TECHNIQUE FOR RIGHT-SIDED TUMOR NEPHRECTOMY

After inspection of the abdominal cavity and positioning of the trocars, access to the retroperitoneum is the

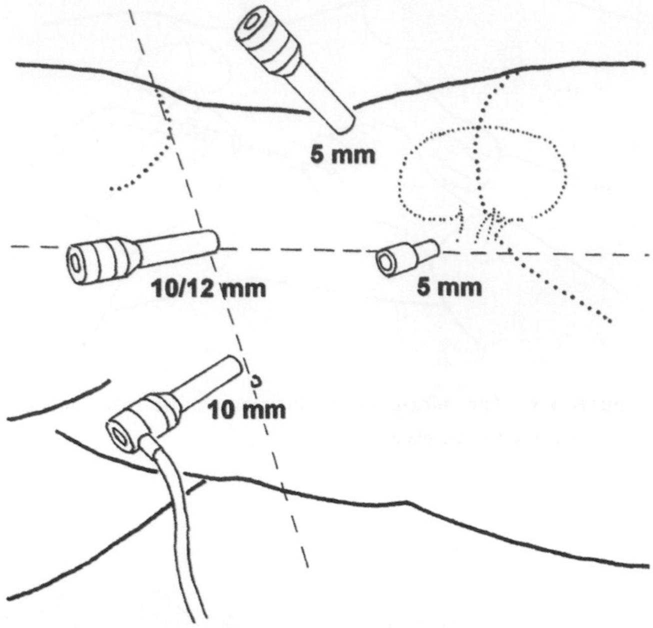

Figure 4.11 Diagrammatic illustration of the four-trocar technique.

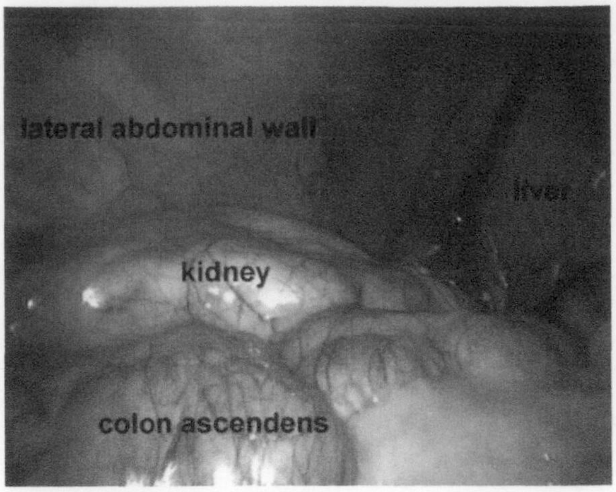

Figure 4.12 This view gives an important anatomic orientation of the right upper abdominal cavity.

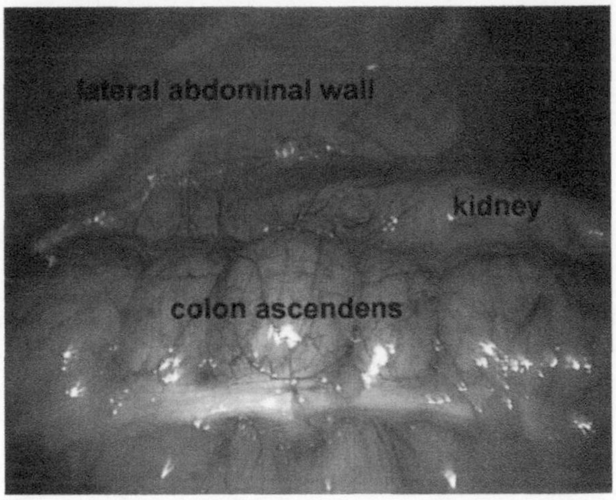

Figure 4.13 The operation starts with the laterocolic preparation of the colon ascendens.

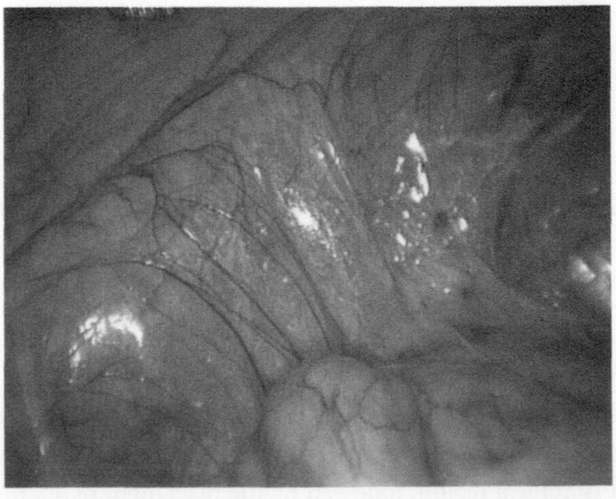

Figure 4.14 If the tissue is pulled back, the tissue layer that has to be incised can be very readily identified.

next step. In some cases, intra-abdominal adhesions have to be resolved. Direct laterocolic preparation can be advised for access to the retroperitoneum. Figures 4.12–4.14 demonstrate the situs of a tumor nephrectomy on the right side with the main anatomic structures.

It is important to identify the layer between mesocolon and kidney by pulling the colon median with a grasper. The transection of the laterocolic tissue should be close to the colon (Figures 4.15 and 4.16). Bipolar coagulation of the tissue is useful to avoid small bleedings that disturb the identification of the anatomic layers during transection.

At this point it is critical to avoid early mobilization of the dorsal aspect of the kidney fat capsule, since the mobilized kidney will dislocate ventrally and the renal hilum cannot be transected under optimal conditions.

There are two principal routes for access to the renal hilum, as described below.

Following colon ascendens mobilization the identification of the ureter at the common iliac vessels is especially recommended for the unexperienced surgeon. Using the ureter as an anatomic landmark it is easy to identify the testicular/ovarian vein, which leads to the vena cava directly below the renal hilum.

Another surgical option is the primary identification and mobilization of the duodenum with access to the inferior vena cava at the junction of the renal vein. Bleeding from duodenal vessels can be controlled with bipolar coagulation.

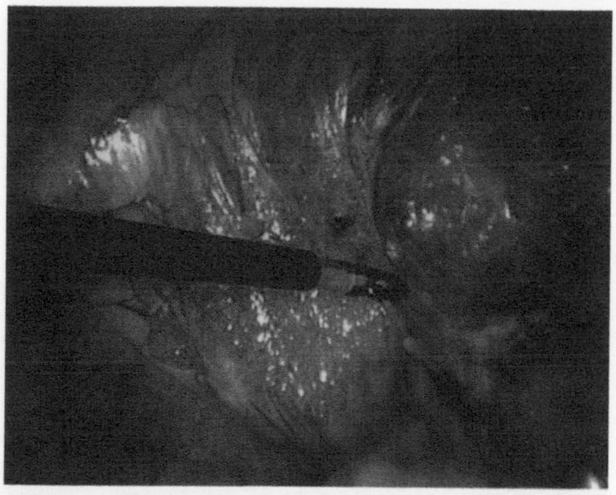

Figure 4.15 Close to the colon, coagulation should be used very carefully. Also, the coagulation of even small bleedings keeps the operating field 'clean', which is helpful for further identification of the tissue layers.

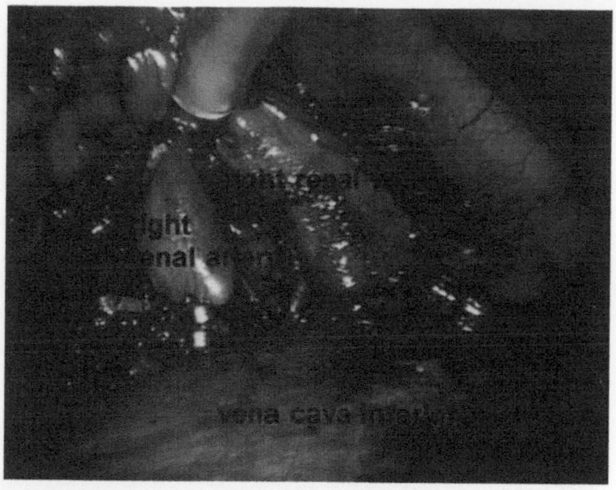

Figure 4.17 This is a view onto the renal hilum of the right side. The artery has to be transected first, therefore, its careful preparation is mandatory.

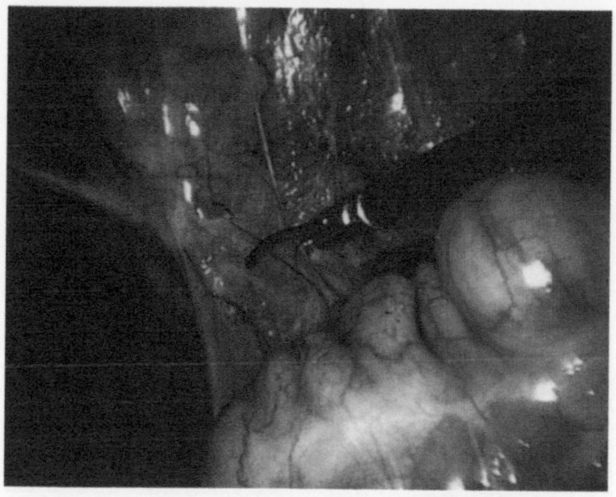

Figure 4.16 When using monopolar coagulation, the surgeon should always make sure that the end of the instrument has no contact with the bowel or other organs.

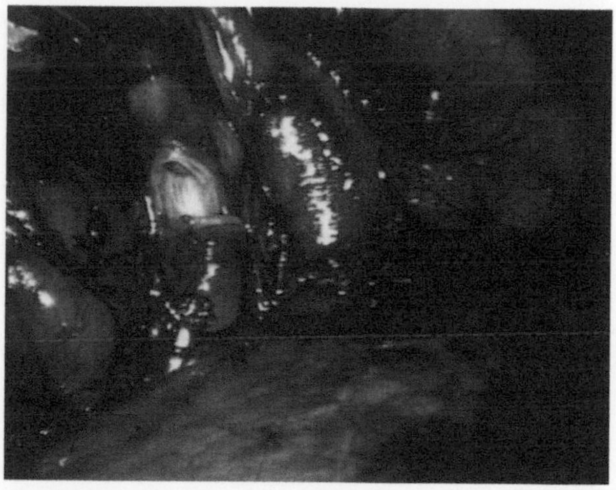

Figure 4.18 The artery can be clipped with titan or Hem-o-lok clips.

The partial lateral preparation of the vena cava is recommended. In some cases, the careful transection of the testicular/ovarian vein might be helpful. We prefer the preparation of the inferior vena cava over a length that equals the kidney. The renal vein and the renal artery will then be identified. In renal tumors on the right kidney, preparation of the lateral vena cava margin cranially to the junction of the liver veins helps in identification of the adrenal vein.

Renal vein preparation is a critical step. Additional renal or lumbal veins should be identified and handled with caution. The use of a 30° camera allows the surgeon to look from above and below the renal vein. With a 10 mm overholt clamp the vein can be separated at the dorsal aspect. Similarly, the preparation of the renal artery can be managed. For the transection of the renal artery non-adsorbable titan clips (Ethicon) or Hem-o-lok clips (Weck) can be used (Figure 4.17). The application of two central clips and one peripheral clip is recommended (Figure 4.18). The renal vein can be secured either by using an Endo-GIA or, as shown in Figures 4.19 and 4.20, by Hem-o-lok clips.

After transection of the renal hilum further preparation of the ureter is recommended. The ureter can easily be transected at the lower pole of the kidney along to the common iliac vessels. Titan clips or Hem-o-lok clips can be used for transection (Figures 4.21 and 4.22).

Starting from the lower pole of the kidney, the compartment can then be further mobilized along the paracaval space to the psoas muscle. At the upper pole the

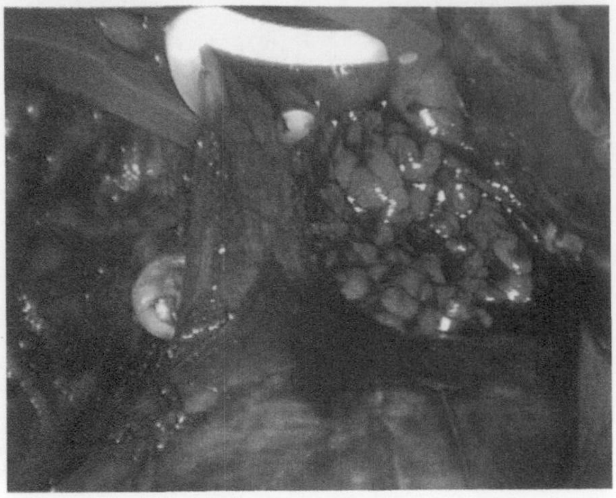

Figure 4.19 The renal vein has to be separated very carefully to avoid damage to this vessel or lumbal veins.

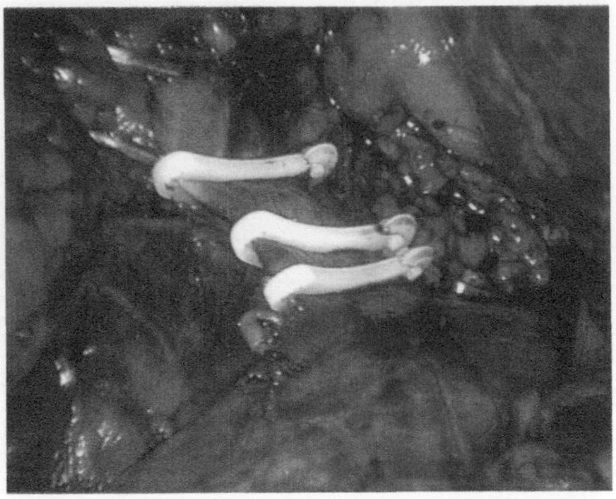

Figure 4.20 In this case, Hem-o-lok clips were used for renal vein transection. An Endo-GIA is also a secure device.

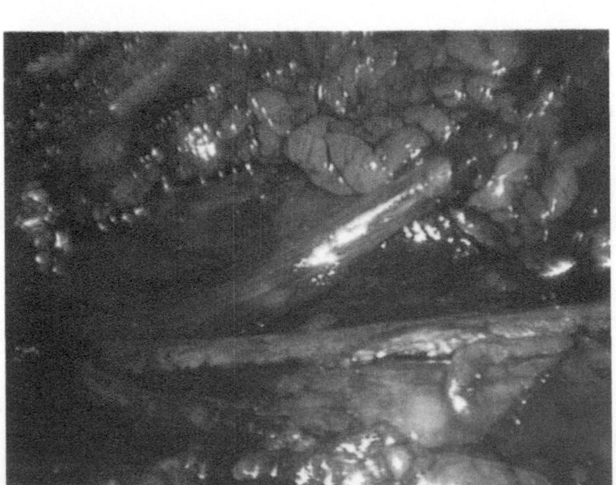

Figure 4.21 If the ureter has already been identified at the beginning of the operation, now time can be saved.

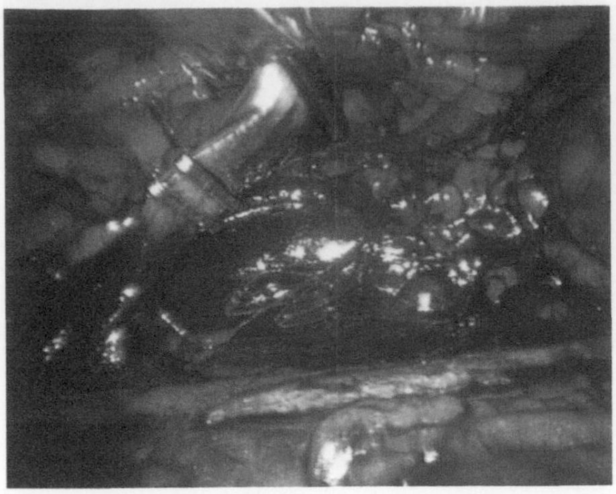

Figure 4.22 The ureter can be transected between titan clips or Hem-o-lok clips.

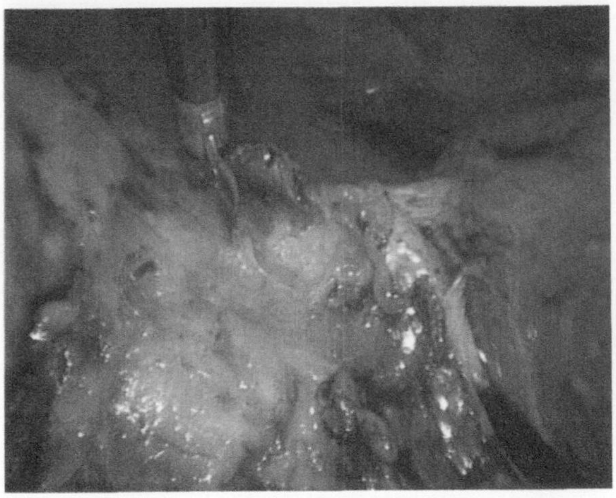

Figure 4.23 The upper pole can be dissected with preservation of the adrenal gland.

transection of the tissue with careful separation of the liver can be challenging (Figure 4.23). Commonly, it is easier to remove the renal compartment with the adrenal gland. In this approach, attention has to be paid to careful transection of the adrenal vein.

If removal of the adrenal gland is not necessary, the renal compartment should be mobilized by direct identification of the medial aspect of the renal capsule from the upper pole of the kidney.

After complete mobilization of the renal compartment with the kidney, the tumor, the fat capsule, and the adrenal gland, preparations for organ retrieval should be made. Several techniques have been reported regarding organ retrieval. We use the lateral 10 mm port for careful insertion of an 10 cm endo-bag. Position of the endo-bag in the direction of the diaphragm is helpful for the

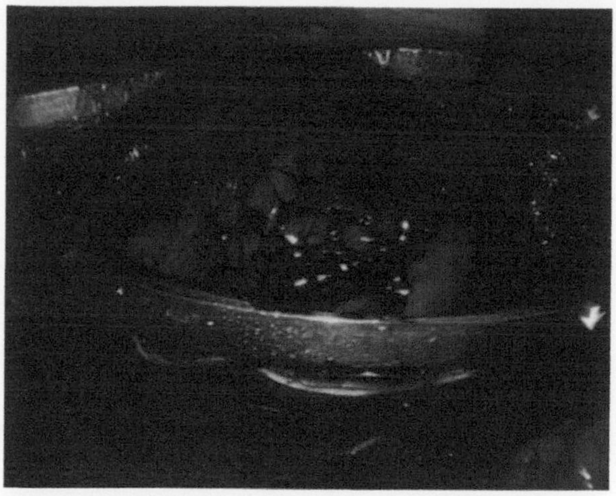

Figure 4.24 The entrapment of the specimen in the LapSac requires careful handling and patience.

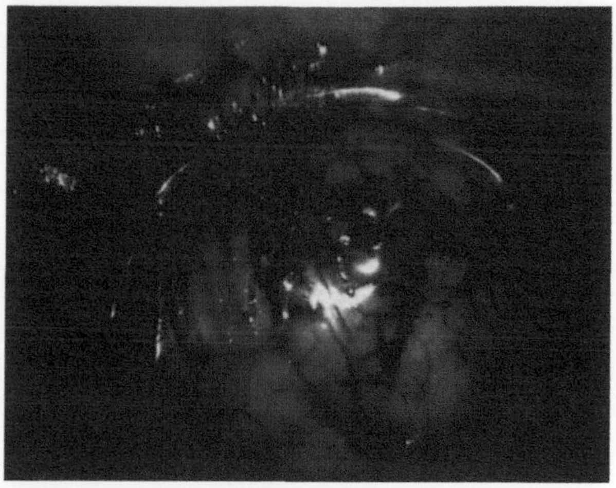

Figure 4.25 If the specimen is entrapped in the bag, it can be retrieved by a muscle-splitting incision.

management of the kidney with its adjacent tissue (Figures 4.24 and 4.25). The movement of the organ specimen into the endo-bag requires experience. Following this procedure the specimen can be retrieved via a 7–8 cm flank incision.

POSTOPERATIVE SCHEDULE

- Fluid intake 2 hours after surgery
- Yoghurt 4 hours after surgery
- Mobilization on the evening of the operation day
- Diet on the first postoperative day
- Regular cost on the second postoperative day
- Pain medication:
  1.5 g methamizole or 1 g paracetamol every 6 hours after surgery
  800 mg ibuprofen twice or 40 drops methamizole/paracetamol at patient's request
- Urinary catheter for 24 hours post surgery.

LITERATURE

CHAPTER 5

Laparoscopic tumor excision – transperitoneal approach

Andreas H Wille

INDICATION

The indication for laparoscopic tumor nephrectomy for small renal masses (< 4 cm) has changed during the last decade and is similar to that for the open approach. To date organ-preserving techniques should always be preferred if possible and the laparoscopic procedure has replaced the open approach in many centers.[1–3]

Renal masses up to 4 cm can be treated with the laparoscopic approach; in some cases even larger tumor masses can resected laparoscopically, depending on the localization. Therefore, indication should be strict and the surgeon should be well experienced with laparoscopic procedures. This chapter describes our technique for laparoscopic partial nephrectomy in warm ischemia with endo-bulldog clamps using a thrombin-gelatin matrix (FloSeal™) for hemostasis.

TECHNIQUE

Basically the laparoscopic technique mimics the steps of open surgery with:

- mobilization of the colon
- preparation of the renal hilum
- mobilization of the renal artery (e.g. renal vein)
- complete mobilization of the kidney and removal of the fatty capsule
- identification of the tumor
- marking of the resection border using monopolar current
- clamping of the renal artery (if necessary) using an endo-bulldog clamp
- resection of the tumor using harmonic or cold scissors
- suturing of defects of the collecting system
- suturing of large vessels
- application of FloSeal™
- removal of the bulldog clamp
- extraction of the specimen via a muscle-splitting mini incision.

Major issues of laparoscopic partial nephrectomy are ischemia and hemostasis. As a bloodless operating field is crucial for proper resection, hilar clamping is advised in most cases. Some very peripherally located tumors do not need ischemia but these are rare. To minimize warm ischema, clamping should be performed at the latest possible moment and tools for suturing and hemostasis must be prepared and ready at this point. Warm ischemia times up to 30 minutes are acceptable but, if necessary, even longer ischemia times can be tolerated without major renal impairment.[4,5]

Different techniques for cold ischemia have been published but their benefits are controversial,[6–8] therefore no standard has been established yet.

Hemostasis may be achieved in different ways with good results. Simple suturing of the defect as in open techniques may be used but, especially for beginners, requires good skills and is time-consuming.[9] Besides, the use of deep parenchymal sutures leads to additional tissue damage, which can be avoided by other techniques. However, modified suturing techniques using oxidized cellulose bolster for compression and different agents for hemostasis are used successfully worldwide.[2,10]

The use of thrombin-gelatin matrix (FloSeal™) has been established in our institution and is used routinely for hemostasis in almost all cases.[11,12]

PREOPERATIVE SCHEDULE

See radical nephrectomy, Chapter 4.

ANESTHETIC REGIMEN

See radical nephrectomy, Chapter 4.

INSTRUMENTATION

- Working port 12 mm
- Working port 10 mm
- Working port 5 mm
- Optical port 10 mm
- Monopolar scissors
- Bipolar forceps
- Ultracision device (optional)
- Atraumatic graspers
- Stump overholt clamp 10 mm
- Endo-bulldog clamps (straight/curved)
- Clamp applicator
- Clamp remover
- Needle driver
- Maryland grasper
- Lahodny™ clip applicator
- FloSeal™ applicator (single use or reusable)
- Lahodny™ sutures 5×0 PDS (curved needle)
- FloSeal™ (one or two vials).

PATIENT POSITION AND PORT PLACEMENT

The position of the patient and the personnel in the operating room are shown in Figure 4.1. Prior to positioning of the patient a transurethral catheter should be placed. We prefer the transperitoneal approach with the four-port technique as used for radical nephrectomy, as described earlier (see Chapter 4). If damage of the collecting system during resection is expected a double-J stent is placed preoperatively. The patient is placed in the extended flank position, the camera port is inserted via an infra-umbilical incision and two additional trocars are placed under direct laparoscopic vision in the mid-axillary line on either side of the first port. After mobilization of the colon a 10 mm port is inserted via a flank incision (see Figure 4.11).

Positioning of the ports is similar to the technique for radical nephrectomy, but, depending on the localization of the tumor, angles for optimal access are different. In cases of dorsal and/or cranial tumors a complete mobilization of the entire kidney is mandatory to maintain accessibility. In such cases principally a more lateral placement of the 12 mm port is advisible for formation of an equilateral triangle between the optical and the working ports.

OPERATIVE TECHNIQUE FOR RIGHT-SIDED PARTIAL NEPHRECTOMY OF A SMALL VENTRAL TUMOR

A 30° optical device should be used to achieve an optimal view for different angles. This is beneficial for the preparation of the renal hilum and also for visualization of the tumor border during the resection. The line of Toldt is incised to reflect the colon medially and dissection proceeds medially until the duodenum is mobilized and the hilum is exposed to gain access to the renal artery. To stay within the proper layers it is important to work strictly between the renal capsule and the colon and use bipolar current for coagulation. Always avoid monopolar current near the bowel and the renal vessels!

If necessary, the renal artery is clamped using endoscopic bulldog clamps (Aesculap-Braun, Tuttlingen, Germany), but resection of small and peripheral lesions could be considered without hilar clamping. First the renal vein has to be visualized and mobilized, using scissors, bipolar forceps, and a stump overhold clamp. This gives proper access to the renal artery and the possibility of clamping if nephrectomy has to be performed in case of an emergency. The partial lateral preparation of the vena cava is recommended. In some cases, the careful transection of the testicular/ovarian vein might be helpful (especially in left-sided tumors). Additional renal or lumbal veins should be identified and handled with caution. After access is achieved, the renal artery has to be mobilized and prepared for clamping. Remember that, in contrast to nephrectomy, the renal vasculature has to be spared during preparation to keep the postoperative perfusion unaffected!

After the hilar preparation is finished the fatty capsule of the kidney has to be removed to visualize the tumor. The grade of mobilization depends on the localization of the tumor. Lower pole tumors possibly require less tissue preparation compared with upper pole or dorsal tumors. However, the mobility of the instruments is limited due to the port position. Therefore the kidney needs mobility to get optimal access to the tumor! Remember, regarding kidney mobilization, more is better!

When the tumor is accessible, a mark around the resection field is set using monopolar current. It is advisable to test the accessibility of the tumor by moving the kidney to find the optimal position for the resection before ischemia is established. At this point mannitol is given intravenously for kidney protection.

After everything is set for resection and hemostasis, including preparation of sutures, FloSeal™, clamp-remover, etc.

(remember: save time as much as you can!), the bulldog clamp is attached to the renal artery.

The kidney is immediately positioned as described earlier and tumor resection is performed with scissors or the harmonic scalpel; in our institution we prefer the latter. Any defects in the pelvicaliceal system are closed with Lahodny sutures in a water-tight fashion. To help identify small lesions blue dye may injected via a preoperatively inserted ureteral catheter or the indwelling Foley catheter if a double-*J* stent has been placed.

We achieve hemostasis exclusively by application of FloSeal™ (Baxter Medical, Fremont, CA, USA).[11] But, if large vessels are affected it might be necessary to place a Lahodny suture in the resection area. The thrombin-gelatin granular matrix has to be applied after resection of the tumor and before reperfusion of the kidney using a special laparoscopy applicator provided by the company. After mixing the two components, it is pushed through the applicator onto the resected surface. Gentle pressure with a moist sponge stick is applied for 1–2 minutes. It is advisable to use the substance sparingly, to retain a little in case of bleeding after clamp removal. For hemostasis a thin layer is sufficient if the resection surface is covered completely. Remember, less is more in this case! After that the clamp has to be removed immediately. The resected tumor must be entrapped in an endo-bag and extracted *in toto* through a small incision mostly performed in the flank involving the lateral port. Frozen sections should be performed in all cases to define tumor integrity and resection margins.

If bleeding is still present an additional application of FloSeal™ may be necessary. Note that the application has to be performed under the primary applied layer to be effective.

Finally the retroperitoneum can be closed with running sutures, but this is not mandatory. For safety a drainage may be inserted, in our institution we do not place a drain routinely.

LAPAROSCOPIC PARTIAL NEPHRECTOMY STEP-BY-STEP

Preparation of the renal hilum is shown in Figures 5.1–5.5.

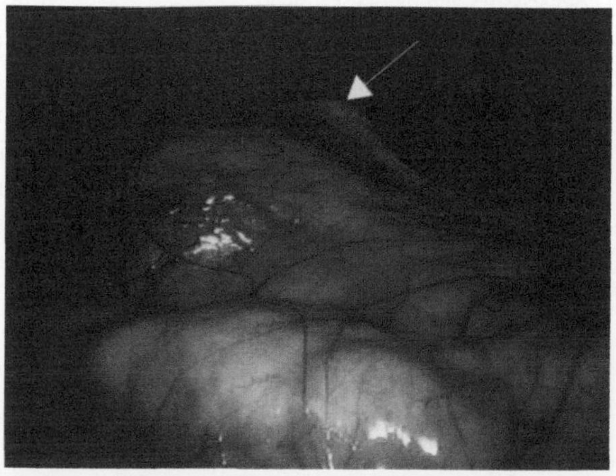

Figure 5.1 Ventrally localized tumor of the right kidney (2 cm).

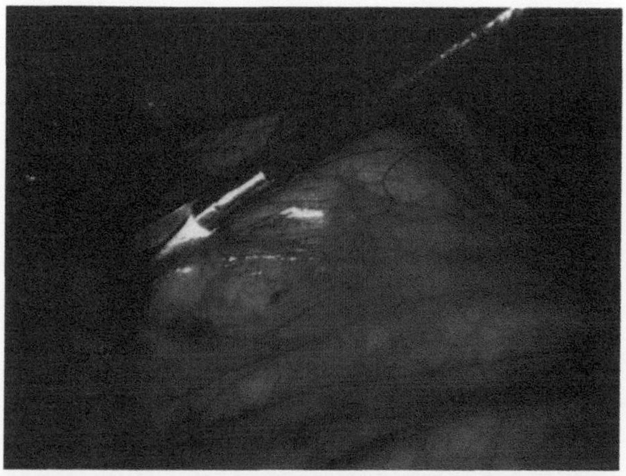

Figure 5.2 Incision of the retroperitoneum and mobilization of the colon ascendens.

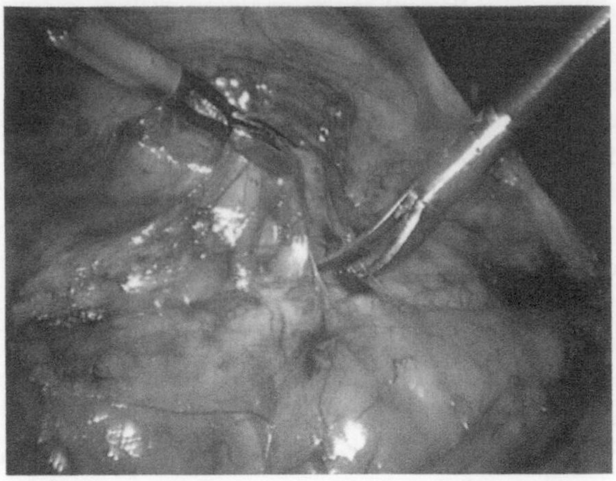

Figure 5.3 Mobilization of the duodenum, the vena cava is going to be exposed.

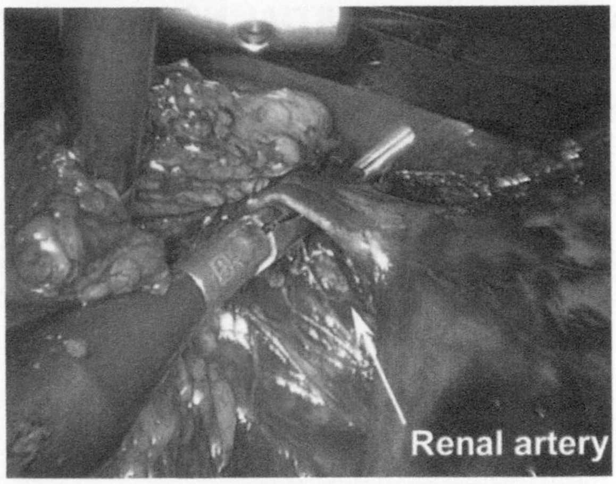

Figure 5.4 Visualization of the renal hilum. The renal vein is mobilized as demonstrated with an overhold clamp.

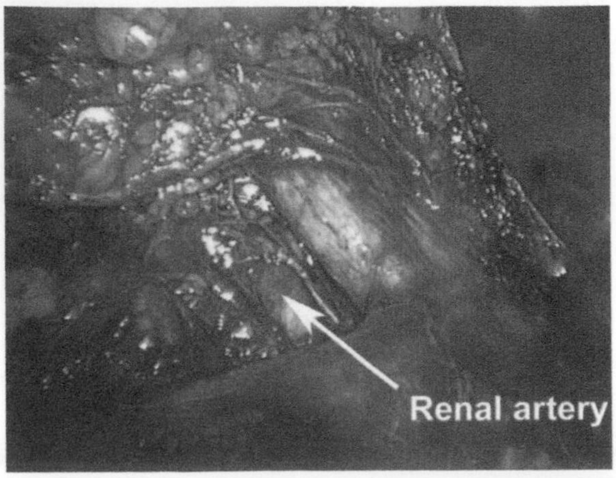

Figure 5.5 After mobilization of the renal vein access to the renal artery is established. Watch out for accessory arteries or branches!

Tumor excision is illustrated in Figures 5.6–5.16.

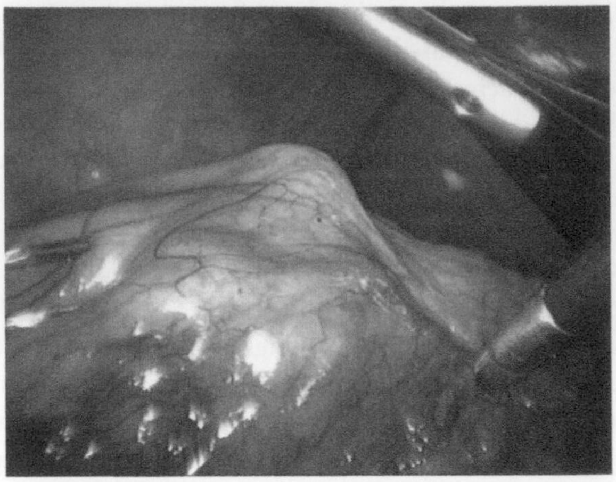

Figure 5.6 Presentation of the tumor, the liver is lifted up with an endo-retractor.

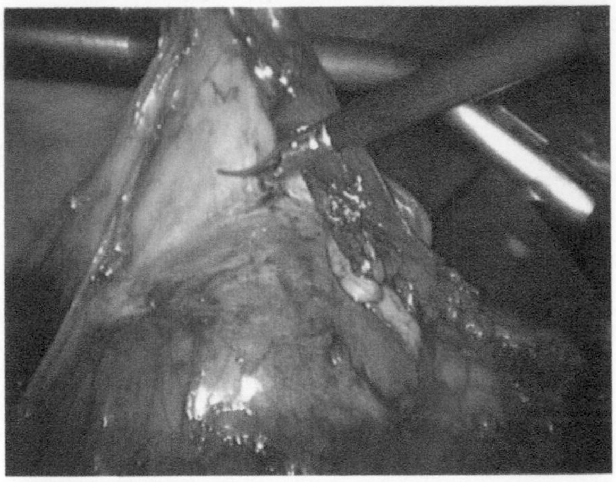

Figure 5.7 Mobilization of the kidney. The fatty tissue is removed using cold scissors and bipolar cautery.

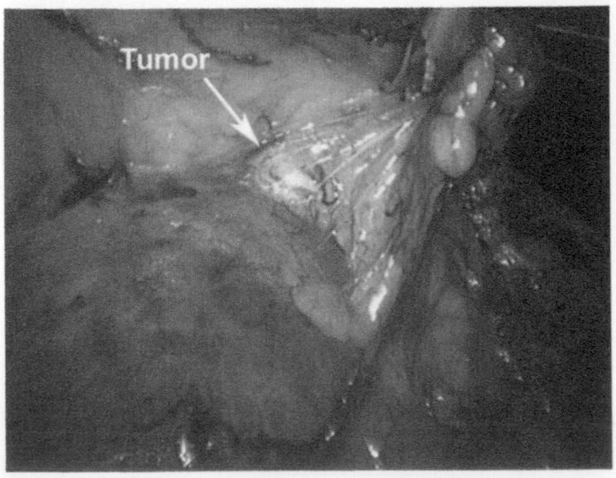

Figure 5.8 The tumor is carefully visualized step by step.

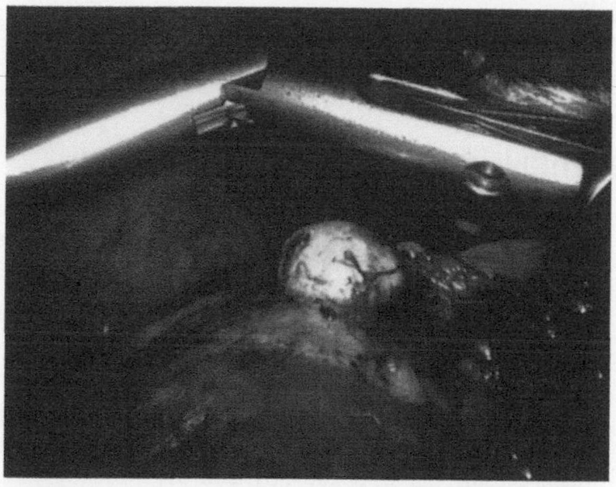

Figure 5.9 The tumor is exposed and the kidney is pushed in the optimized position for resection.

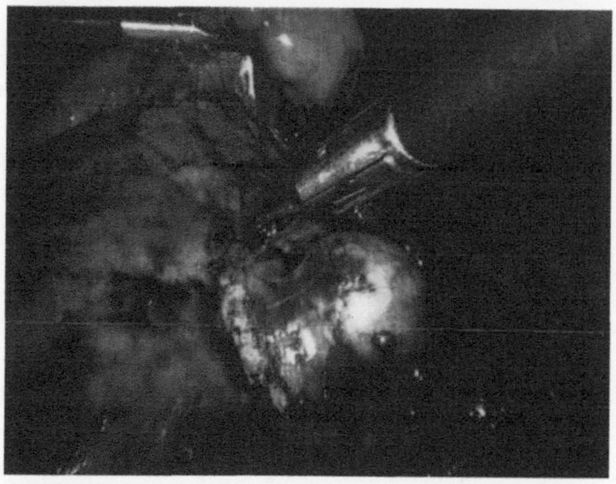

Figure 5.10 Marking of the resection border using monopolar current.

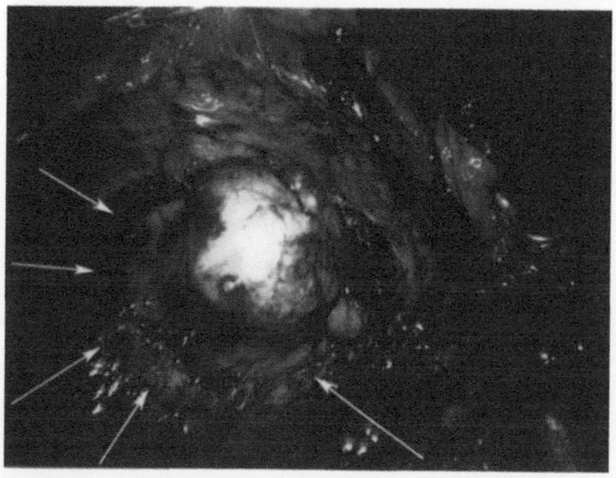

Figure 5.11 The tumor is circumferentially marked and the capsula fibrosa is incised.

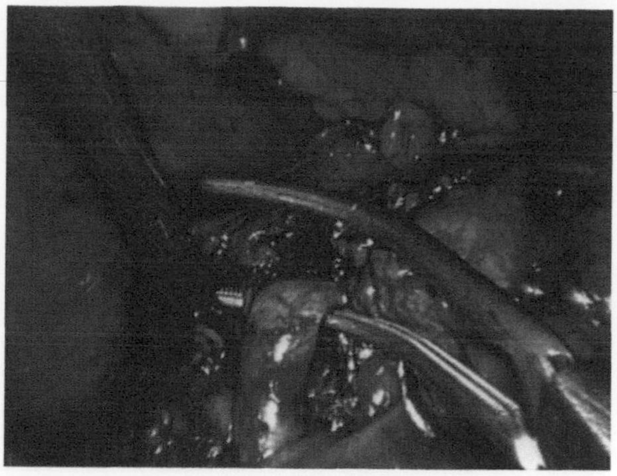

Figure 5.12 Application of the endo-bulldog clamp.

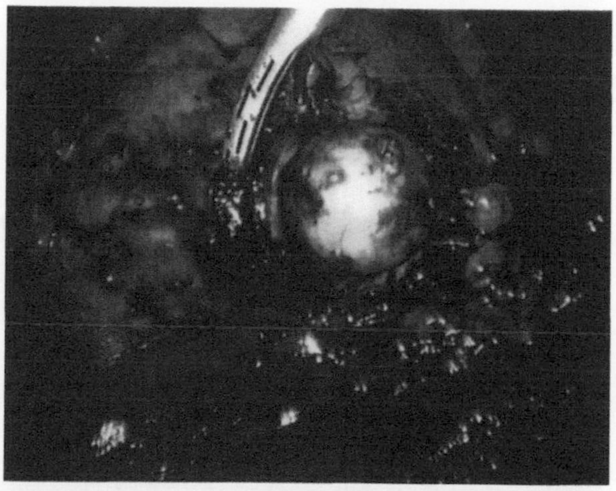

Figure 5.13 Resection of the tumor along the marked line using the UltraCision™ device.

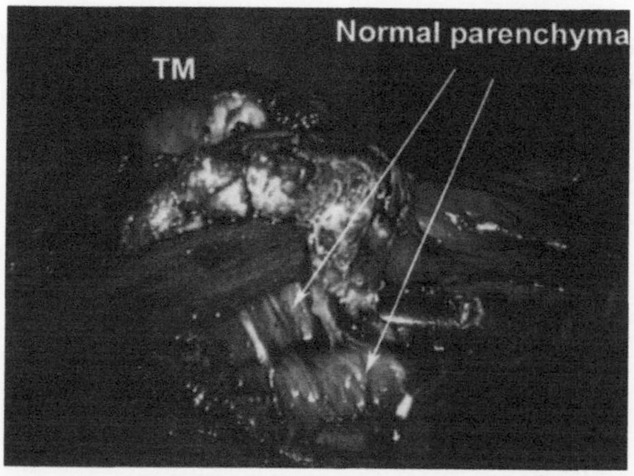

Figure 5.14 Resection continues. Mobilization can be performed partly in a stump fashion as in open procedures. TM, tumor.

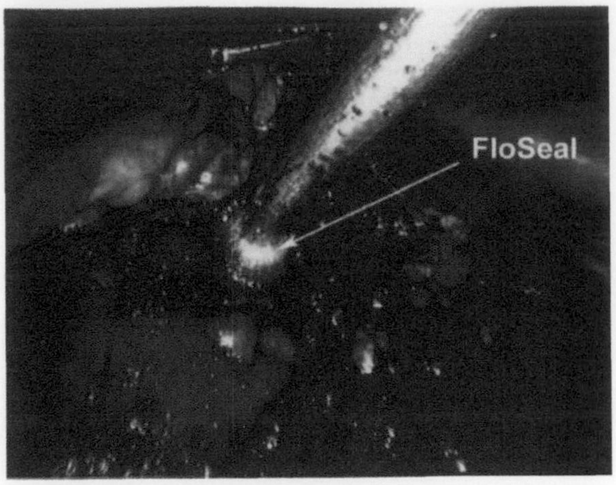

Figure 5.15 Application of FloSeal™ using a customized metal applicator.

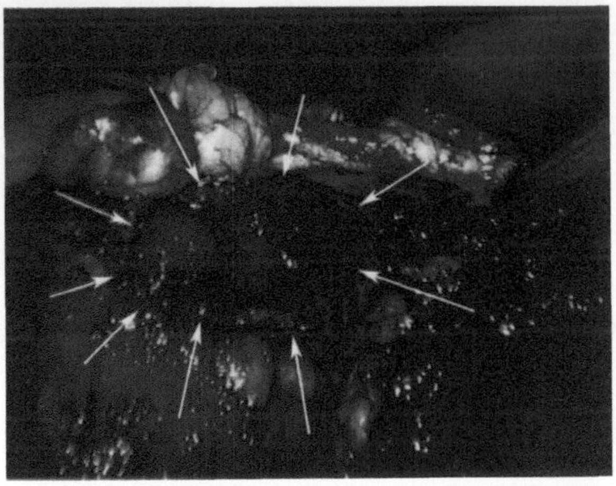

Figure 5.16 Final situation after removing the bulldog clamp. No additional hemostasis is necessary.

POSTOPERATIVE SCHEDULE

See tumor nephrectomy, in Chapter 4.

REFERENCES

1. Martorana G, Bertaccini A, Concetti S et al. Nephron-sparing surgery for renal cell carcinoma: state of the art and 10 years of multicentric experience. Eur Urol Suppl 2006; 5: 600–9.
2. Häcker A, Albadour A, Jauker W et al. Nephron-sparing surgery for renal tumours: acceleration and facilitation of the laparoscopic technique. Eur Urol 2007; 51: 358–65.
3. Aron M, Gill IS. Minimally invasive nephron-sparing surgery (MINSS) for renal tumours. Part I: laparoscopic partial nephrectomy. Eur Urol 2007; 51: 348–57.
4. Sherkarriz B, Shah G, Upadhyay J. Impact of temporary hilar clamping during laparoscopic partial nephrectomy on postoperative renal function: a prospective study. J Urol 2004; 172: 54–7.
5. Desai MM, Gill IS, Ramani AP et al. The impact of warm ischaemia on renal function after laparoscopic partial nephrectomy. BJU Int 2005; 95: 377–83.
6. Landman J, Venkatesh R, Lee D et al. Renal hypothermia achieved by retrograde endoscopic cold saline perfusion: technique and initial clinical application. Urology 2003; 61: 1023–5.
7. Janetschek G, Abdelmaksoud A, Bagheri F et al. Laparoscopic partial nephrectomy in cold ischemia: renal artery perfusion. J Urol 2004; 171: 68–71.
8. Gill IS, Abreu SC, Desai MM et al. Laparoscopic ice slush renal hypothermia for partial nephrectomy: the initial experience. J Urol 2003; 170: 52–6.
9. Desai MM, Gill IS, Kaouk JH, Martin SF, Novick AC. Laparoscopic partial nephrectomy with suture repair of the pelvicaliceal system. Urology 2003; 61: 99–104.
10. Klingler CH, Remzi M, Marberger M, Janetschek G. Hemostasis in laparoscopy. Eur Urol 2006; 50: 948–57.
11. Wille AH, Tüllmann M, Roigas J, Loening SA, Deger S. Laparoscopic partial nephrectomy in renal cell cancer – results and reproducibility by different surgeons in a high volume laparoscopic center. Eur Urol 2006; 49: 337–43.
12. Richter F, Schnorr D, Deger S et al. Improvement of hemostasis in open and laparoscopically performed partial nephrectomy using a gelatine matrix-thrombin tissue sealant (FloSeal). Urology 2003; 61: 73–7.

CHAPTER 6

Retroperitoneoscopic living donor nephrectomy

Alexander Bachmann and Robin Ruszat

INDICATION

Typically, a living donor is either an immediate blood-related family member or a spouse of the recipient who has end-stage renal failure. Recently, altruistic third-party donation has gained considerable attention. All potential donors are routinely evaluated according to a donation protocol. Their suitability is discussed in detail by the transplantation team comprising nephrologist, urologist, visceral and vascular surgeon, transplantation coordinators, immunological laboratories, and psychosomatic experts. Preoperatively, contrast-enhanced magnet resonance angiography (MRA) is performed to evaluate the vascular anatomy in all donors. The left kidney is preferred for donor nephrectomy because of the longer left renal vein, which facilitates the implantation process. There is consensus that the 'better' kidney should always remain with the donor, so that in case of certain anatomic conditions such as multiple arteries, venous anomalies, vascular stenosis or an early arterial branching the right kidney needs to be harvested.

PREOPERATIVE SCHEDULE

The patient is admitted to hospital 1 day before surgery and undergoes routine preoperative evaluation including blood analysis, chest X-ray, and electrocardiography. Special bowel preparation is not necessary for retroperitoneoscopy. In order to prevent thombosis the patient receives subcutaneous low-molecular-weight heparin on the evening before the operation. One hour preoperatively broad-spectrum antibiotics are administered intravenously. Following general anesthesia and Foley catheter placement, the patient is safely secured to the operating table in a standard full-flank position.

STEP-BY-STEP OPERATIVE TECHNIQUE

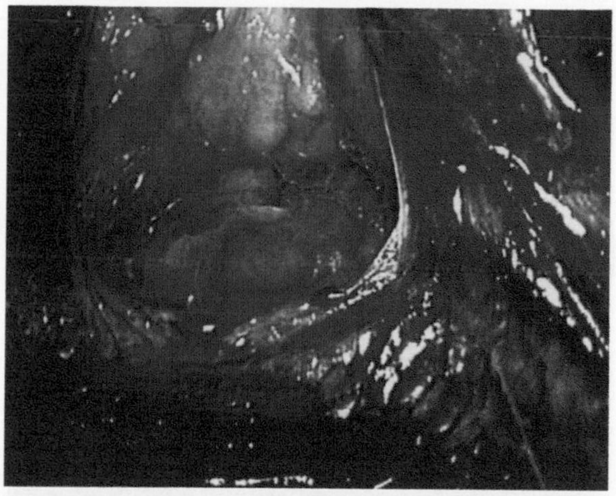

Figure 6.1 The dissection starts with horizontal incision of the Gerota's fascia, which lies above and parallel to the psoas muscle. It is important to perform the incision over the entire length of the fascia to obtain a large working space. It is necessary to leave the anterior fixation of the kidney to the peritoneum, which guarantees enough space and good overview for vessel preparation. In donor nephrectomy, an additional fourth trocar is mandatory. With this, a clamp is inserted over the fourth trocar and can be used to hold the kidney more ventrally.

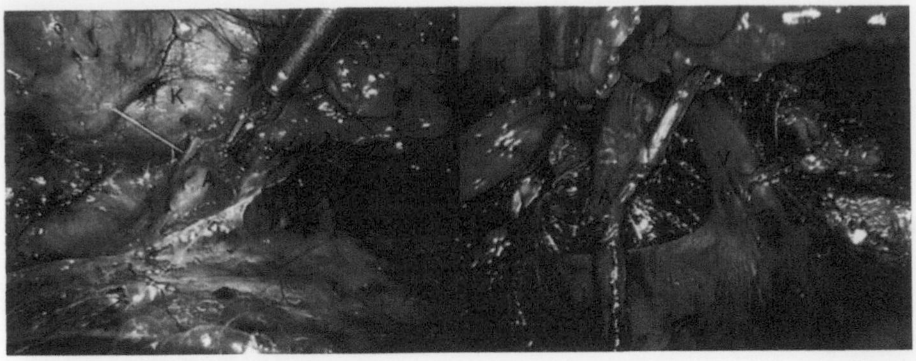

Figure 6.2 After the Gerota's fascia is incised the renal hilum can be identified very easily and surrounding fatty and connective tissue is dissected carefully from the renal vessels using the tip of the suction device, bipolar forceps, and scissors. The renal artery (A) can easily be identified by its pulsating appearance. It is necessary to free the renal vessels as completely as possible from the surrounding tissue. Perihilar and perivascular lymph nodes and lymphatics must be severed and coagulated in the course of this process. Excessive coagulation must be avoided under any circumstances owing to the thermal damage to the renal vessels that this entails. In contrast, excessive application of clips to ligate blood vessels and lymphatics is disadvantageous for the planned renal vessel resection. Characteristically, the left renal hilus is surrounded by well developed lymphatics that not uncommonly open directly into a cisterna chyli or variably into a lymphatic plexus. Iatrogenic injury should be treated directly with small clips, bipolar cautery, or if possible, direct stitching with 4-0 monofilm sutures. V, renal vein, K, kidney.

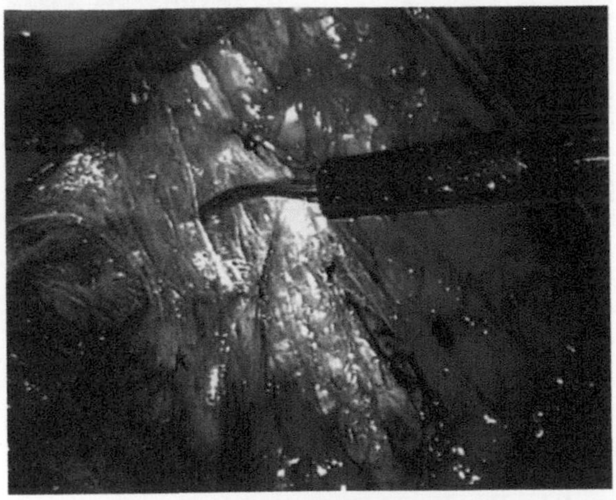

Figure 6.3 After careful dissection of the renal vessels is completed, the kidney (K) is usually bluntly freed from connective tissue using monopolar and bipolar cautery. In cases where there has been pyelolithotomy or kidney inflammation the step can be difficult and time-consuming. Care has to be taken at the upper kidney pole where the adrenal gland is located. P, peritoneum.

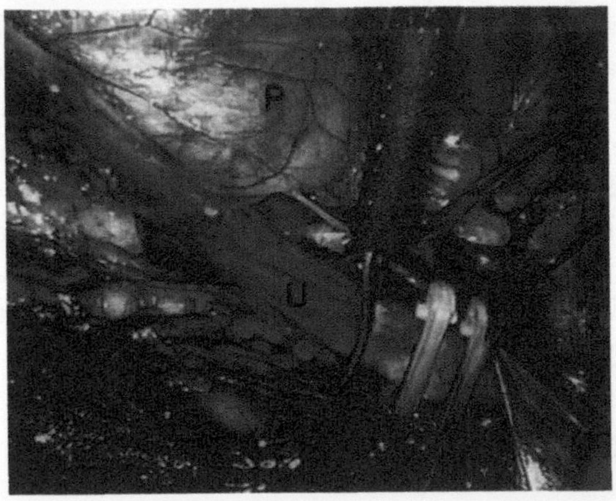

Figure 6.4 The ureter (U) is identified and carefully prepared caudally. It is important not to dissect surrounding fatty tissue that is essential for ureteral perfusion. Usually the ureter is transected in the region where the ureters' vessels cross. Absorbable clips can be used. P, peritoneum.

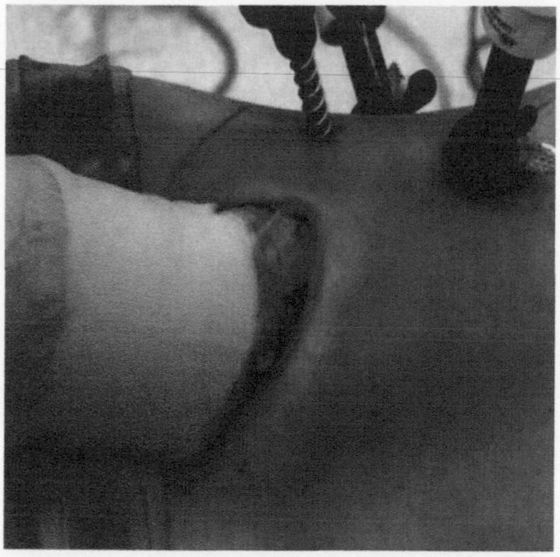

Figure 6.5 Harvesting of the kidney is performed with manual assistance. For this purpose, the lower trocar access is enlarged up to 7–9 cm by a muscle split incision and the surgeon's hand is inserted directly into the retroperitoneum. The incision diameter should be large enough to ensure a safe, quick, and careful removal of the kidney.

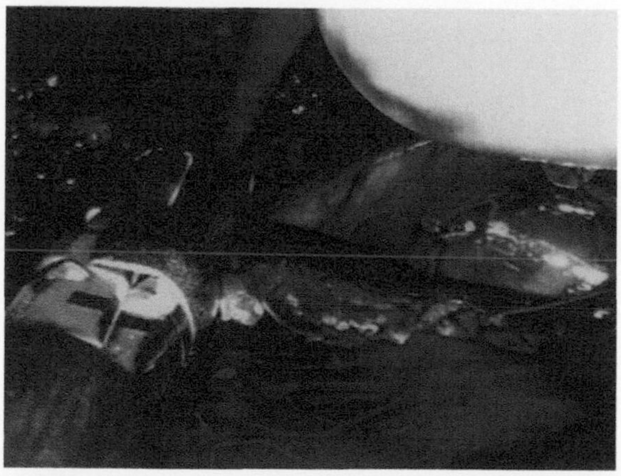

Figure 6.6 For vessel transection we prefer to use a TA-30-2.5 (AutoSuture®) disposable stapler for both artery and vein. It provides an additional 2–3 mm length of the right graft vein, compared with the commonly used Endo-GIA™ stapler. The stapler is pushed down and the artery and vein are pulled up to obtain the maximum length of both vessels.

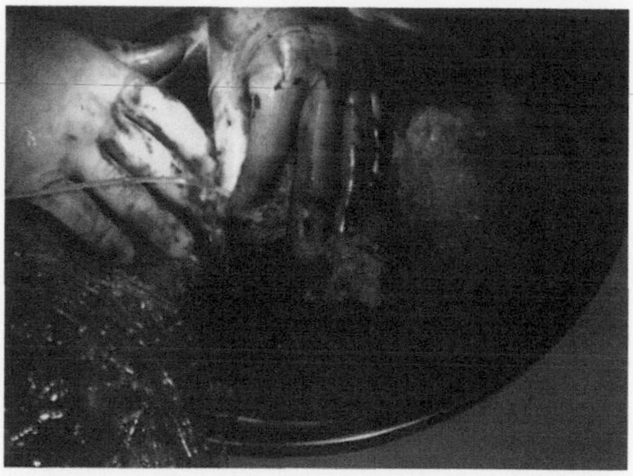

Figure 6.7 After the kidney is harvested it is directly laid in crushed ice and perfused with cold storage solution (Viaspan®) until a clear effluvium is visible from the vein. Afterwards, the kidney is put in a sterile plastic bag and taken straight to the next theater room, where the implantation is performed immediately.

CHAPTER 7

Laparoscopic donor nephrectomy – transperitoneal approach

Serdar Deger

INDICATION

The indication is a wish to make a kidney donation.

PREOPERATIVE SCHEDULE

The preoperative schedule is the same as for laparoscopic nephrectomy (see Chapter 4).

INSTRUMENTATION

The instrumentation is the same as for laparoscopic nephrectomy (see Chapter 4). The exception is an endoscopic Satinsky clamp for right-sided donor nephrectomy.

STEP-BY-STEP OPERATIVE TECHNIQUE

The positioning of the patient, surgeons, and nurse in the operation room are the same as for laparoscopic nephrectomy (see Figure 4.1). The position of the patient on the operation table is the same as for laparoscopic nephrectomy (see Figure 4.2). The position of the trocars for the operation field is also the same as for laparoscopic nephrectomy (see Figure 4.11).

The access and bowel preparation are as same as laparoscopic nephrectomy (see Chapter 4).

Right side

The renal vein has to be prepared on the right side from the inferior vena cava. Until the renal hilum, the inferior vena cava must be mobilized 2 cm above the renal vein and down to the gonadal vein. Normally the right-sided renal artery is long enough and the inferior vena cava can be rotated as in a right-sided retroperitoneal lymphadenectomy. In these cases the renal artery can be clipped under the inferior vena cava.

We routinely put two central clips and leave the kidney side unclipped regarding reducing warm ischemia time, because this allows easier access to the artery for perfusion intubation and crushing the arterial intima. In cases with early bifurcation or multiple arteries an intra-aortocaval preparation of these vessels in full length is mandatory (Figure 7.1). All clips have to be removed during the *in vitro* preparation of the donated kidney. Therefore there should be enough space on vessels for suturing after clip removal.

A small incision is made medial to the right anterior superior iliac spine, and an endoscopic Satinsky clamp (Satinsky atraumatic clamp, AESCULAP, Tuttlingen, Germany) is inserted into the peritoneum under direct vision (Figure 7.3a). This instrument is

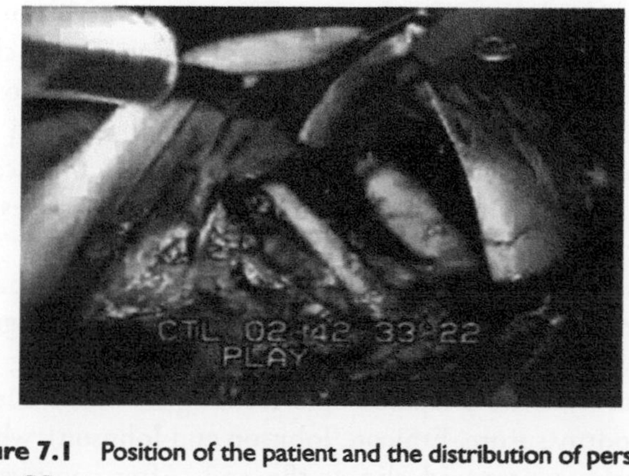

Figure 7.1 Position of the patient and the distribution of personnel in the OR..

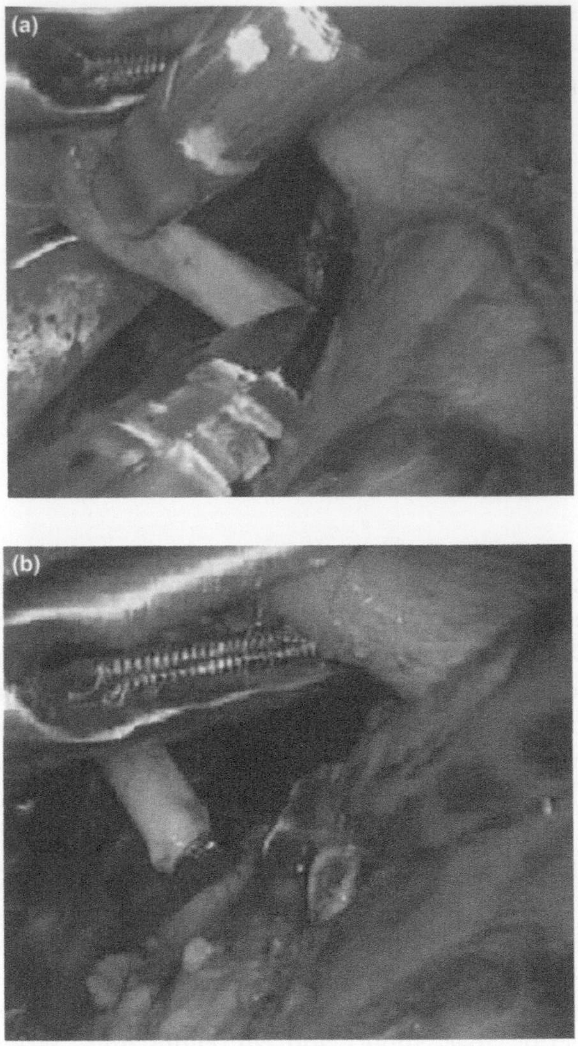

Figure 7.2 (a) Clipping the right renal artery under the inferior vena cava. (b) Central clipping only.

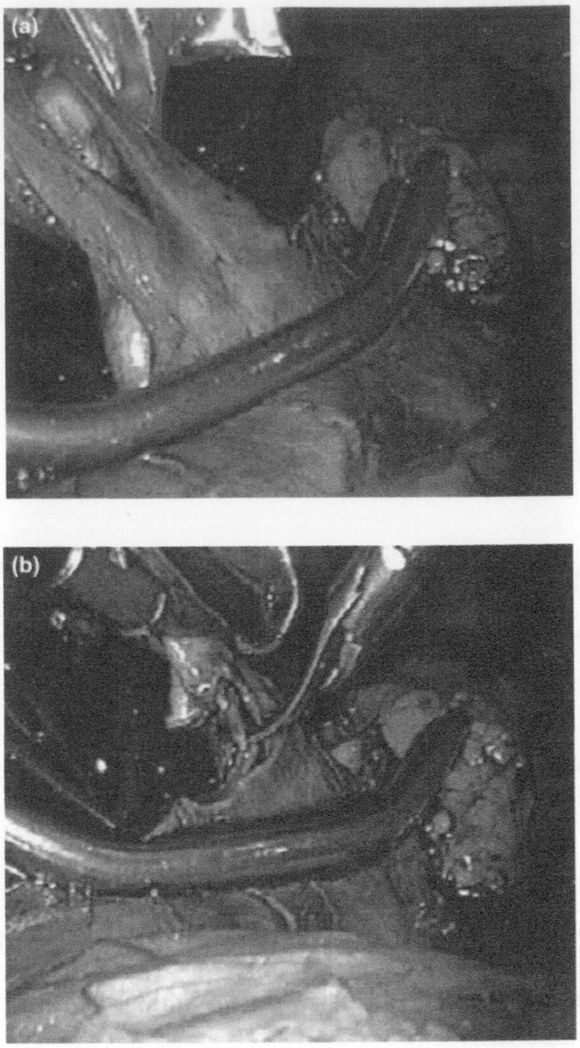

Figure 7.3 (a) Placement of an endoscopic Satinsky clamp on the right renal vein. (b) Cutting the right renal vein.

inserted without a trocar to allow full flexibility for positioning at the inferior vena cava. The vena cava is clamped, and the renal vein is transected sharply using scissors close to the cava (Figure 7.3b). Then the endo-bag is closed, the peritoneum incised, and the bag removed with the kidney and provided to the perfusion team. In these cases warm ischemia time is reduced because no staple lines are present that need removal.

The donor extraction site is closed with absorbable sutures, and the pneumoperitoneum is established again. The vascular clamp can be removed after closing the cavotomy with a laparoscopic running 3-0 PDS suture (Lahodtny suture, Ethicon, Johnson and Johnson), which includes a prepared clip at the end. After completing a running suture a PDS clip is placed to avoid tying. (See Figures 7.4–7.8.)

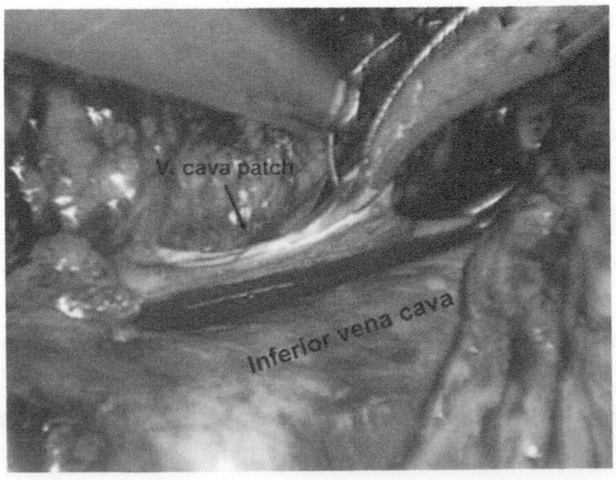

Figure 7.4 Closing of the patch of the inferior vena cava side.

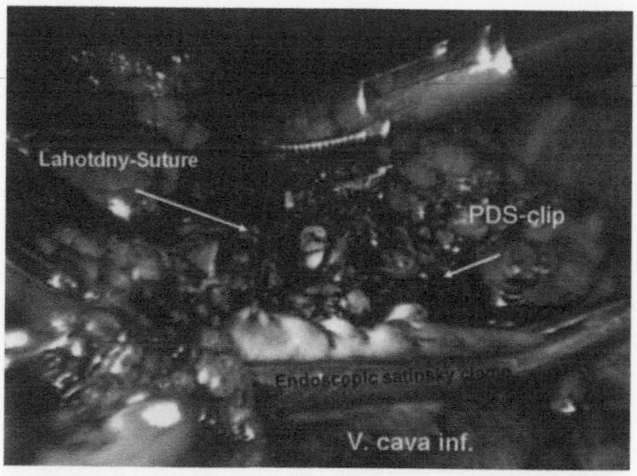

Figure 7.5 Closing the inferior vena cava using 3×0 PDS running suture.

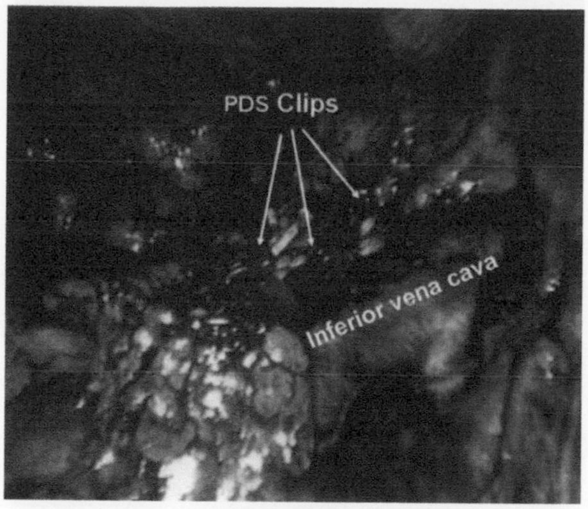

Figure 7.6 Situs after Satinsky clamp removal.

Left side

The left vein has to be clarified completely, gonadal, suprarenal, and lumbal veins must prepared and double-clipped (Figure 7.7). After the whole mobilization of the left renal vein, the left renal artery can be identified easily and prepared – beginning from the aorta until enough space for a central double-clipping is achieved. (See Figures 7.7–7.10.)

After putting the kidney into an endo-bag as described in the harvesting section and retraction, the artery is divided first as shown Figure 7.11. The left vein can be closed and divided using a vascular stapler (Figure 7.12).

The rows of the stapler have to be removed afterwards by the perfusion team.

Harvesting

The kidney has to be mobilized completely until the kidney is only attached to the vessels. A detachable specimen bag is placed through a lateral port site separated from the applicator, and the kidney is placed inside (Figure 7.13).

The organ needs to be introduced into the endo-bag completely (Figure 7.14). The kidney can retracted with the bag (Figure 7.15).

The lateral trocar incision is then enlarged 5–6 cm for organ extraction. The fascia and muscle layers are divided, but the peritoneum is left intact to maintain insufflation. When the kidney vessels are severed, the peritoneum can be opened and retracted from the prepared incision. After the separation of vessels the peritoneum is opened, and the bag is removed with the kidney and provided to the perfusion team.

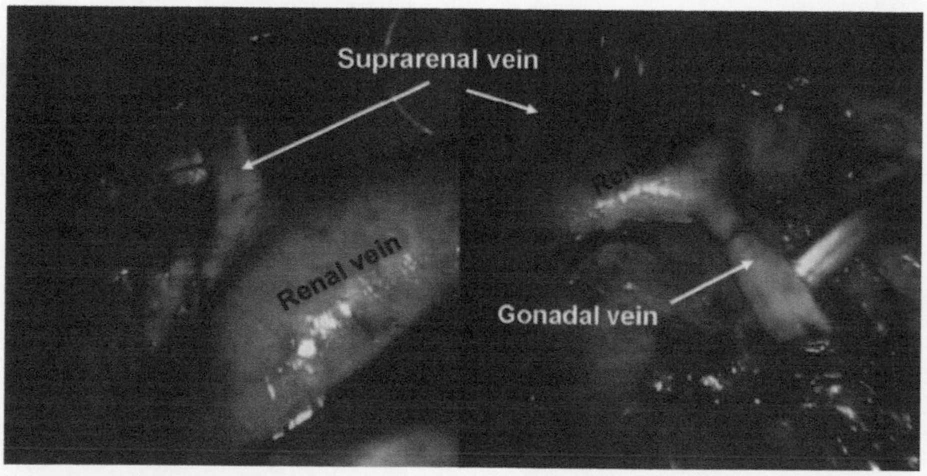

Figure 7.7 Clarifying the left vein completely.

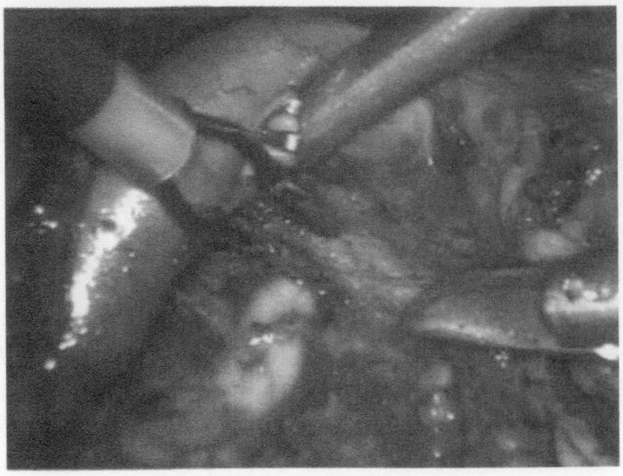

Figure 7.8 Reaching the left artery from the aorta.

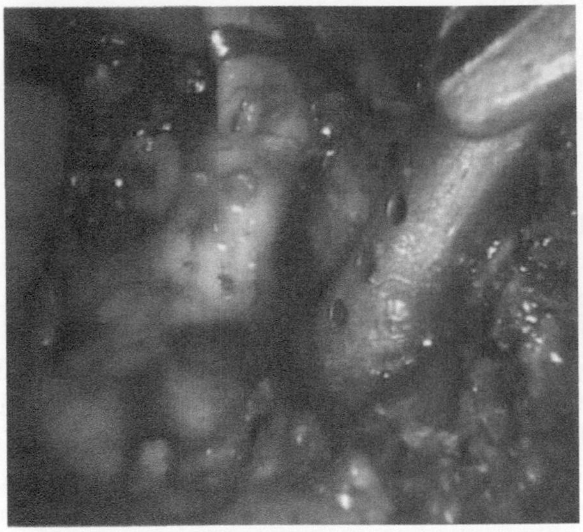

Figure 7.9 Aortal identification.

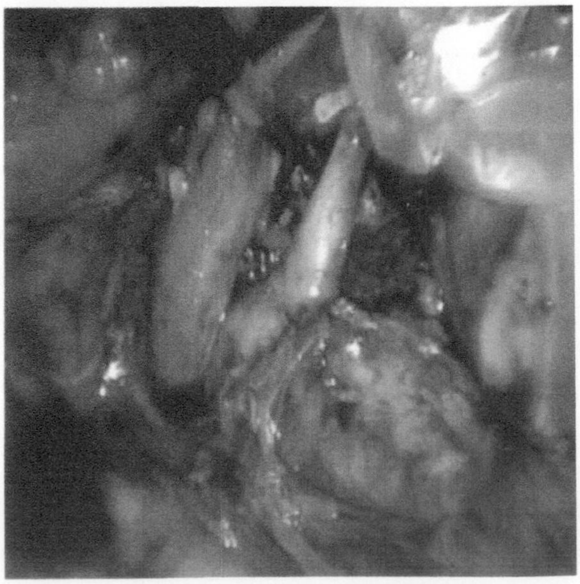

Figure 7.10 Completed preparation of vein and artery.

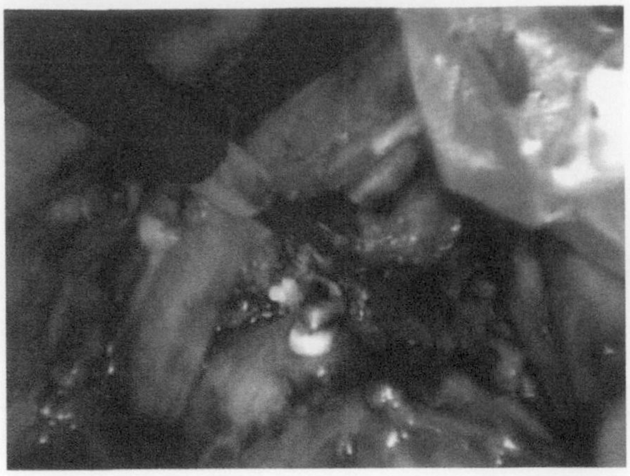

Figure 7.11 Central clipping and separation of the artery.

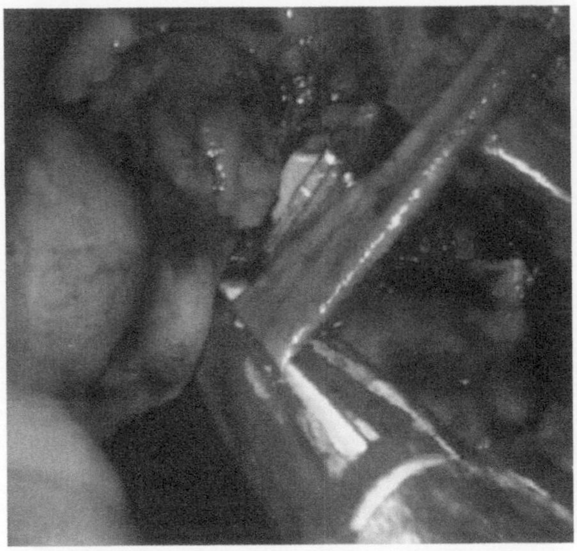

Figure 7.12 Using a vascular stapler for the left renal vein.

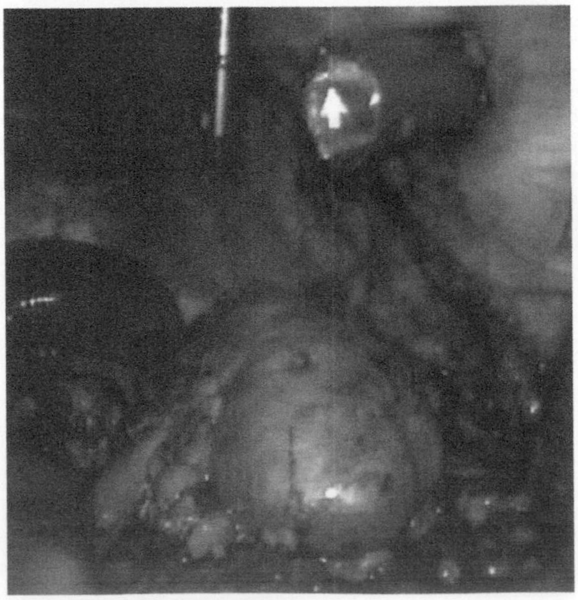

Figure 7.13 Introducing the endo-bag into the abdomen.

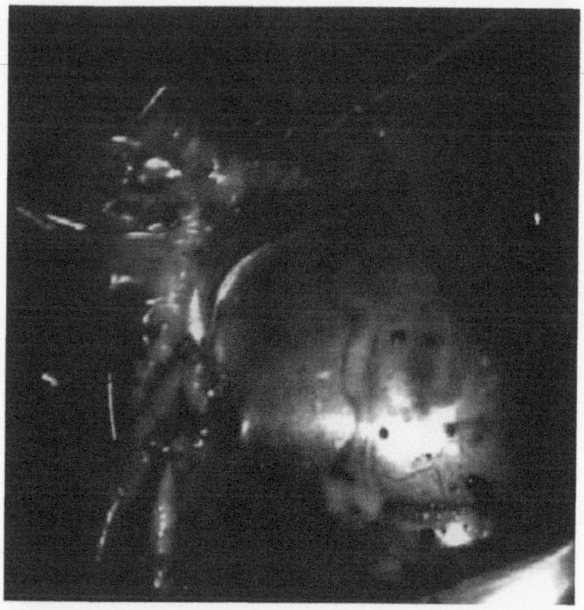

Figure 7.14 Complete covering of the endobag intracorporeally.

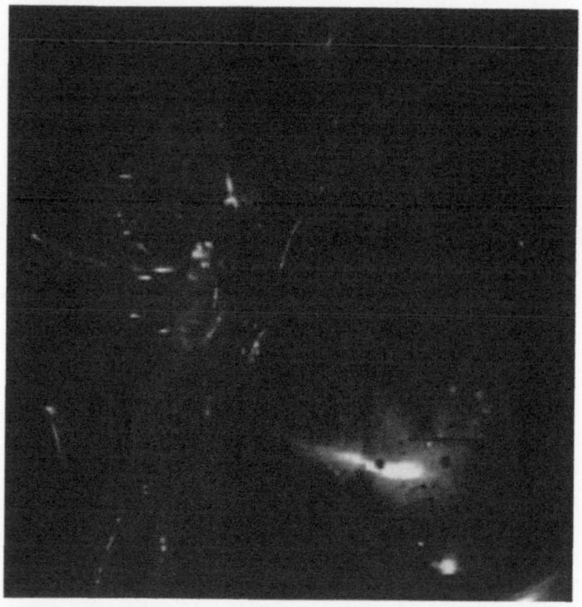

Figure 7.15 Traction of the kidney using an endo-bag.

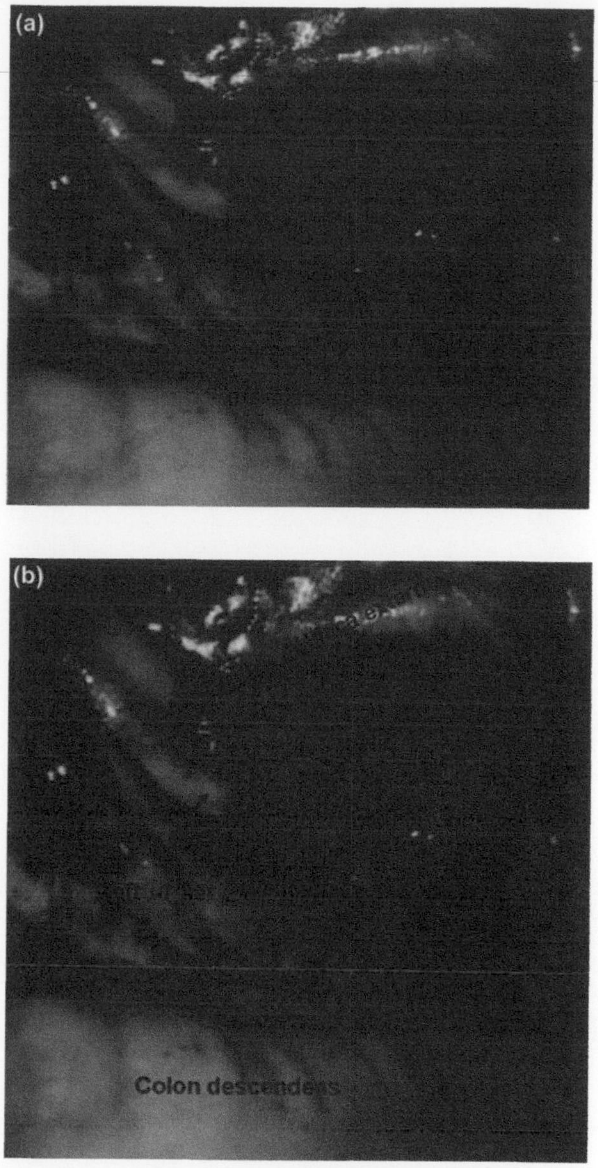

Figure 7.16 Ureter mobilization below iliacal junction.

Ureteral preparation

The ureter should be mobilized in a non-touch technique. The fat tissue around the ureter should not be compromised, small vessels to the ureter must be clipped, thermal damage due to any coagulation must be avoided. The ureter should be mobilized below the iliacal junction (Figure 7.16).

CHAPTER 8

Laparoscopic pyeloplasty

Jan Roigas

INDICATION

Laparoscopic pyeloplasty was first described by Schuessler et al. in 1993.[1] Since then, the laparoscopic approach has become more and more accepted and, currently, this technique is not only commonly used in adult urologic surgery but also for the treatment of children with a ureteropelvic junction obstruction.[2,3]

Pyeloplasty is an operation for the experienced laparoscopic surgeon, since it requires accurate tissue preparation with preservation of lower pole vessels and perfect application of intracorporeal suturing techniques.

Different techniques have been published for the intraoperative management of ureteropelvic pathology. These techniques principally mimic the open surgical approach.[2,4,5] The retroperitoneoscopic and transperitoneal laparoscopic approaches have been published.[2,6,7] The retroperitoneoscopic technique avoids opening the peritoneal cavity for a procedure that is strictly performed in the retroperitoneal space by open surgery. On the other hand, the transperitoneal laparoscopic technique allows an excellent preparation of the retroperitoneal space, an optimal view, and enough room for intracorporel suturing. It is our opinion that, especially for the less experienced laparoscopic surgeon, the transperitoneal laparoscopic route should be employed. At our hospital we prefer the transperitoneal laparoscopic dismembered Anderson-Hynes procedure.[2] In recent years robotic assisted laparoscopic pyeloplasty using the da Vinci or Zeus robotic systems has gained increasing interest.[8–10]

The indication for laparoscopic pyeloplasty is similar to that for open surgery. Obese patients or patients with previous surgery represent no contraindication. In children, this method has been shown in small patient series to be feasible in very young infants of less than 2 or even 1 year of age.[11,12] This operation can also be successfully performed when previous treatment approaches such as endopyelotomy and open or even laparoscopic pyeloplasty have failed.[13]

The indication for laparoscopic pyeloplasty is similar to that for open surgery and mainly relies on the occurrence of urinary tract infections, recurrent flank pain, reduced renal function and impaired.

Prior treatment of the ureteropelvic junction is not necessarily a contraindication for laparoscopic surgery.

The placement of sufficient perioperative drainage of the renal pelvis is still a matter of discussion. We tend to place a double-J-stent and a catheter before surgery. This has the disadvantage that the pelvis is not filled with urine, which renders its preparation more difficult. The placement of a percutaneous nephrostomy is another possibility for sufficient drainage. However, this may have a negative impact on the patient's postoperative quality of life. On the other hand, it allows ease of testing the ureteropelvic junction after suturing for extravasation of a dye. Also, the intraoperative laparoscopic insertion of a double-J stent over the incised ureteral stump has been described and currently seems to be the most accepted solution.[14,15] This technique is feasible but requires careful attention to ensure that the stent is definitely positioned in the urinary bladder.

PREOPERATIVE SCHEDULE

- Diet: Patients can have a normal breakfast in the morning, soup for lunch, and fluid only in the evening.
- Bowel preparation: No specific bowel preparation is necessary. Two rectal enemas are administered in the evening.
- Perioperative antibiotic treatment: Third-generation cephalosporin is used as a single shot during surgery and should be given orally for 3 days postoperatively.

INSTRUMENTATION

- 1 trocar (10 mm)
- 1 trocar (5 mm or 10 mm)
- 1 trocar (5 mm)
- 1 trocar (5 mm) optional
- Optical system (10 mm, 30°)
- Scissor with monopolar coagulation, grasper, overhold clamp, needle holder, bipolar grasper
- 5×0 vicryl with a ct1 needle (optional 6×0 vicryl) for running sutures.

POSITIONING OF THE PATIENT/ OPERATIVE TECHNIQUE

Figure 8.1 demonstrates the positioning of the patient and the medical staff in the operating room. Before positioning the patient a transurethral catheter should be placed in the urinary bladder. Then the patient is placed on his healthy side into a lateral decubitus position. The kidney to be operated on should be lifted up at a 45° angle (Figures 8.2 and 8.3).

The further steps for successful establishment of the pneumoperitoneum are described in Chapter 4 on tumor nephrectomy. Briefly, the table is flexed away from the surgeon, then the patient will be moved in a head down position. At that point the infra-umbilical incision can be made and the Veress needle can be placed. Three trocars have to be placed. Beside the 10 mm, 30° optical trocar at the infra-umbilical site, one 5 mm trocar has to be placed under visual control in the pararectal region on the left side in the middle of the line between umbilicus and spina iliaca anterior superior. Similarly, on the upper pararectal side, a second 5 mm trocar should be placed (Figure 8.4). An optional 5 mm trocar can be placed in the flank.

After all trocars have been placed the peritoneal cavity should be inspected. Then the access to the retroperitoneal space should be started with laterocolic incision of the peritoneum along the line of Toldt. For a right-sided pyeloplasty the cecum and colon ascendens have to be removed and placed medially. Here, it is useful to localize the ureter slightly above its crossing with common iliac vessels. After this preparation the duodenum needs to be identified and mobilized. At this point the vena cava with the junction of the renal vein can be seen in most cases. Usually no further preparation is necessary and the surgeon can begin with the identification and preparation of the upper ureter, the ureteropelvic junction and the pelvis.

For a left-sided pyeloplasty, after the mobilization of colon descendens and the colon sigmoideum, similar to the right side, the ureter should be identified above the

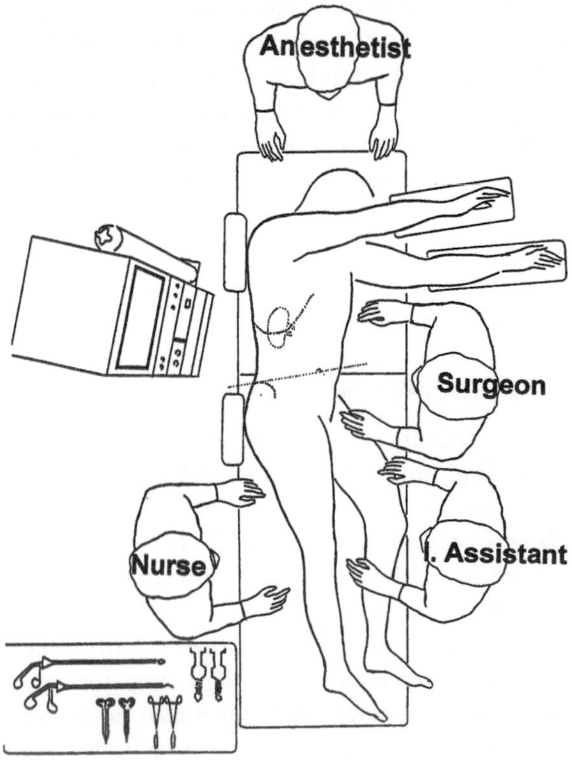

Figure 8.1 Operating room with position of the patient and the personnel.

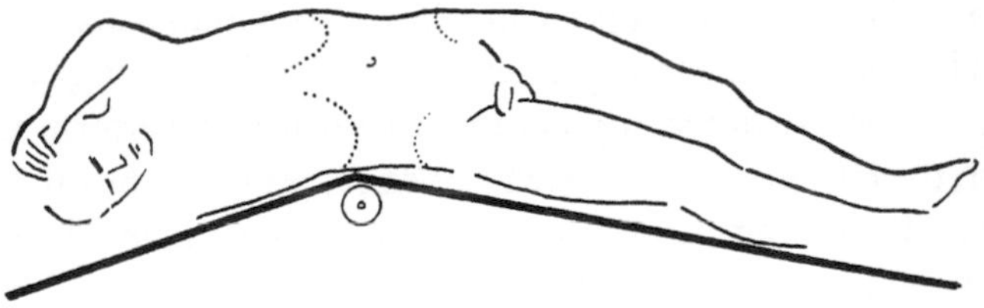

Figure 8.2 Patient is positioned in a flexed manner of the healthy side.

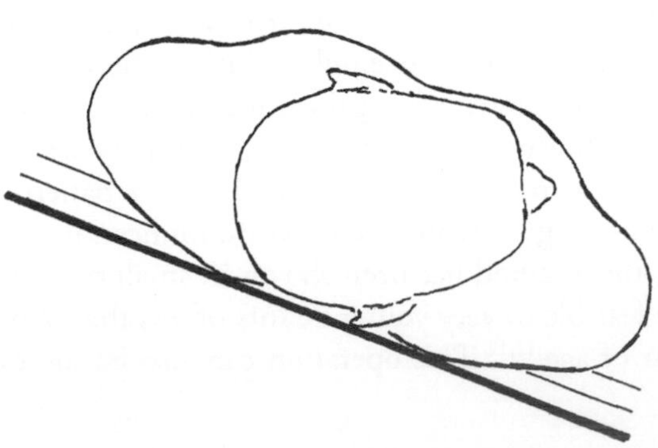

Figure 8.3 The patient is lifted up for about 45°.

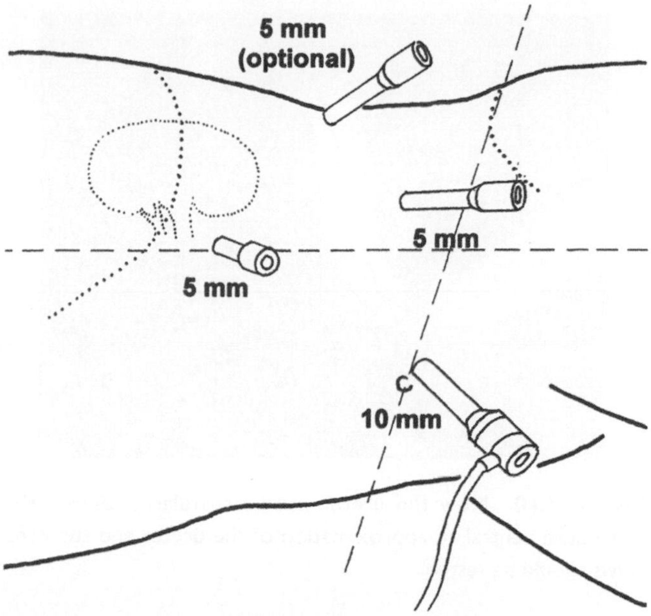

Figure 8.4 Trocar placement with a 10 mm optic trocar, and two 5 mm pararectal trocars. A 5 mm trocar in the flank is optional.

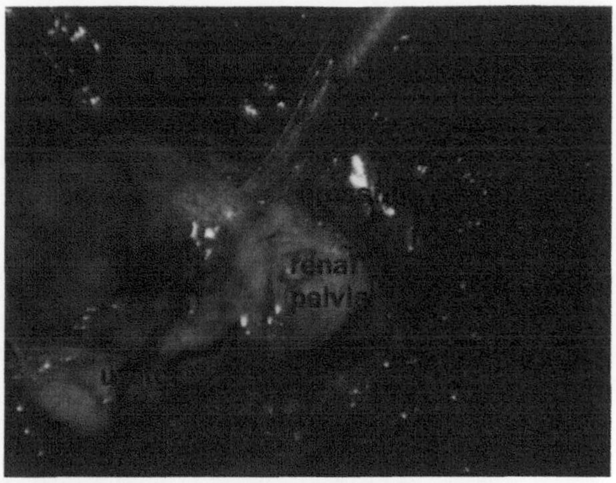

Figure 8.5 After laterocolic preparation and identification of the ureter the ureteropelvic junction should be identified. In this case, a crossing vessel can be seen.

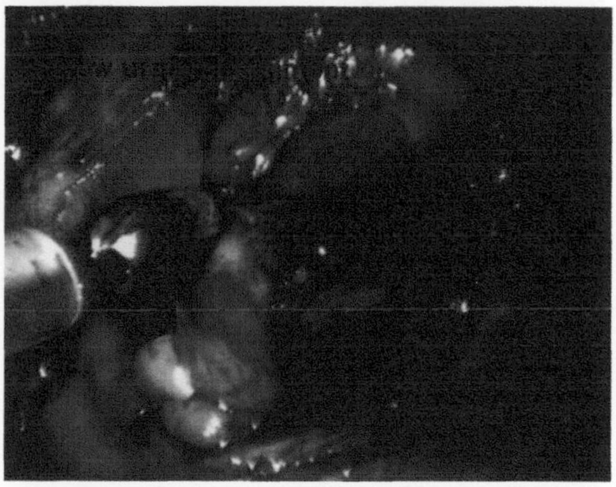

Figure 8.6 The narrow ureteral segment was adherent to the crossing vessel.

crossing with the common iliac vessels. Usually, it is not necessary to mobilize the spleen because a good separation of the colon descendens allows the preparation of the upper ureter and the renal pelvis.

The transmesocolic approach is another means of access to the renal pelvis. This technique is especially useful in children and thin adults on the left side, when the anatomic structures can be easily identified.[16]

During careful preparation of the upper ureter the cause of the ureteropelvic junction obstruction can be seen. In our own patient series, we have found crossing vessels in about 70% of the cases (Figure 8.5). The further preparation of the tissue should be very careful, the lower pole vessels have to be kept intact. Very often, the narrow section at the ureteral insertion can be noticed (Figure 8.6). The mobilization of the upper ureter and the renal pelvis is critical at this point to gain enough length for further reconstruction. If both ends are too short, mobilization of the lower pole of the kidney or even the complete kidney can help to approximate the ends of these structures. On the other hand, the ureter should not be separated completely over a long distance from surrounding tissue to avoid scarring due to reduced blood supply.

Now the ureteroplevic junction can be transected (Figure 8.7). The double-J stent can be identified after incision of the pelvis (Figure 8.8). The ureter is separated and prepared for spatulation (Figure 8.9). As in open surgery, the ureteral tissue should look healthy, otherwise the proximal end should be resected and sent to pathology. The spatulation of the ureter is not easy (Figure 8.10). Here the extact assistance can be very helpful. Now the renal pelvis can be resected if necessary. The resection of renal pelvis under laparoscopic view requires experience and should be done very carefully.

After spatulation of the ureter, resection of remal pelvis, and re-approximation of ureter and renal pelvis, the first two 'anchor' sutures should be inserted at the ventral aspect of the crossing vessels and at the deepest point of the renal pelvis (Figure 8.11). We use absorbable 5×0 vicryl with a ct1 needle as a running suture. Shortening the length of the suture to 12–14 cm can be recommended, because that makes the handling of the sutures much easier. For tying the knots of the first no anchor

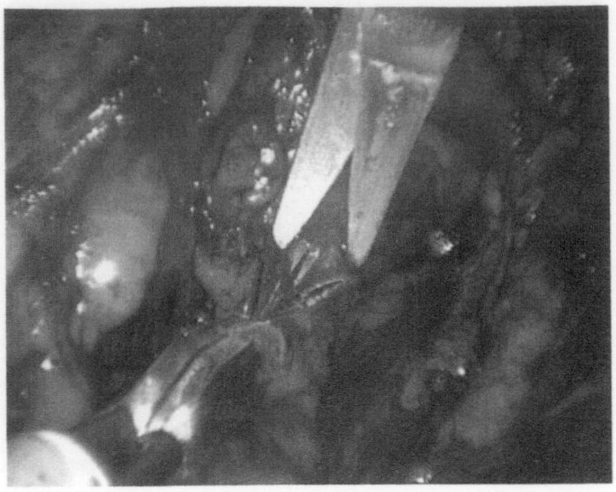

Figure 8.7 When the renal pelvis and the upper ureter have been mobilized the ureteropelvic junction can be transected.

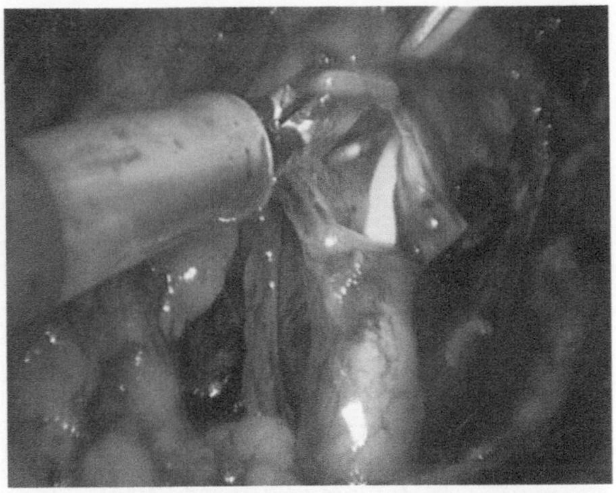

Figure 8.8 The orthotopic double-J stent can be identified in the renal pelvis, which can be resected, if necessary.

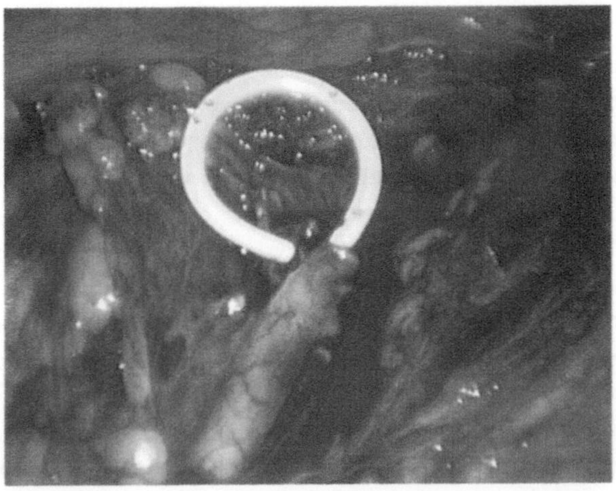

Figure 8.9 When the renal pelvis and ureter are dismembered, attention should be paid to dislocation of the stent.

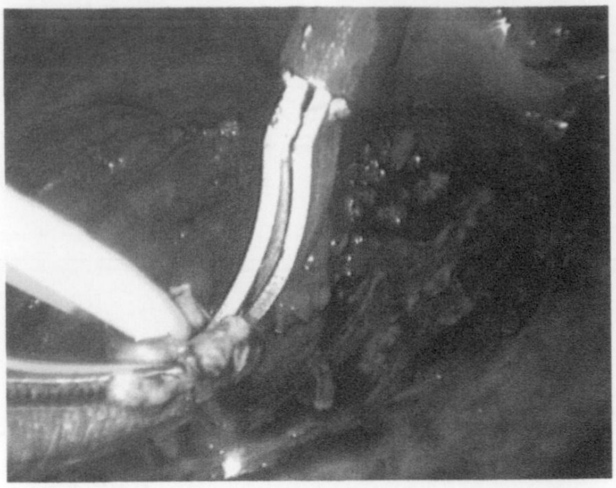

Figure 8.10 Now the ureter can be spatulated. Before this procedure ventral re-approximation of the ureter and the renal pelvis should be tested.

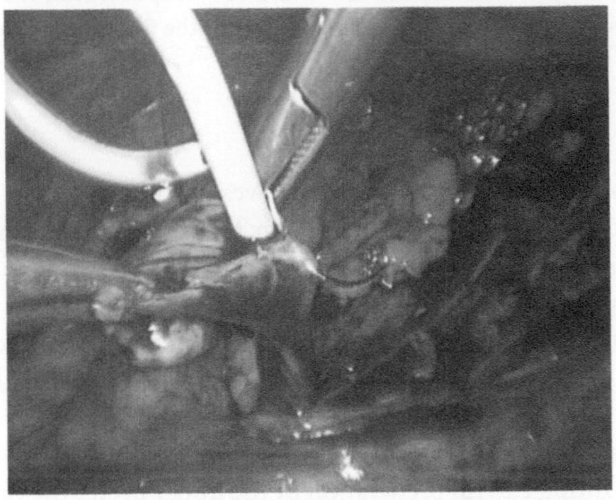

Figure 8.11 The first anchor stitch can be done from outside-in with a 5×0 vicryl suture and a rb-1 needle.

sutures, deflexing the patient may be helpful for careful approximation of the ureteral and pelvic end (Figure 8.12). After successfully tying these knots and insertion of the double-J stent into the renal pelvis, a ventral and dorsal running suture should be performed (Figures 8.13–8.16). If the renal pelvis was resected, a third running suture has to be used for the closure of the pelvis, starting cranially and going distally to the two other sutures. At the end, after performing three or four transverse sutures, all three stitches should be tied to each other. The anastomosis should be inspected for leakage (Figure 8.17). If necessary additional sutures can be inserted. There are various different ways to test the anastomosis for a leakage. If the patient has a percutaneous nephrostomy, then the application of a dye (methylene blue or indigo carmine) provides sufficient evidence of a leakage. Another way is the

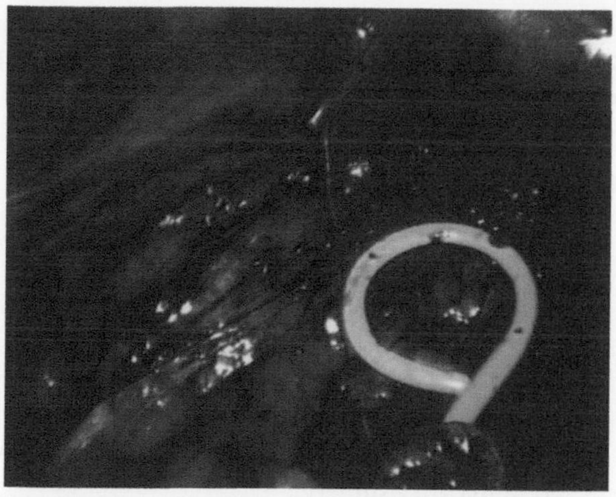

Figure 8.12 The two knots for the anchor stitches should be tied very carefully; sometimes is it is useful if the assistant helps to approximate the tissue with a grasper.

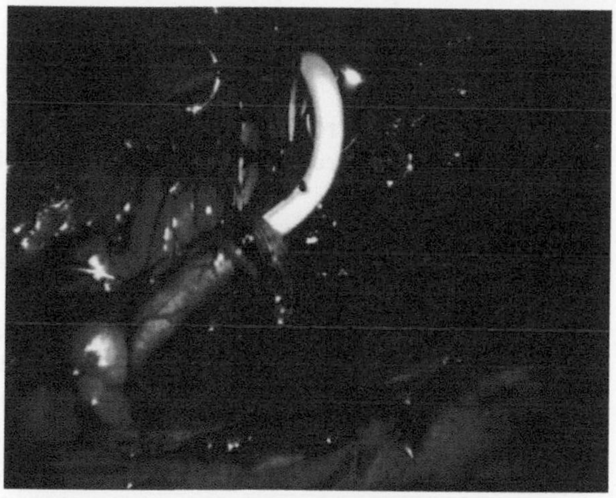

Figure 8.13 Now the double-J stent should placed into the renal pelvis.

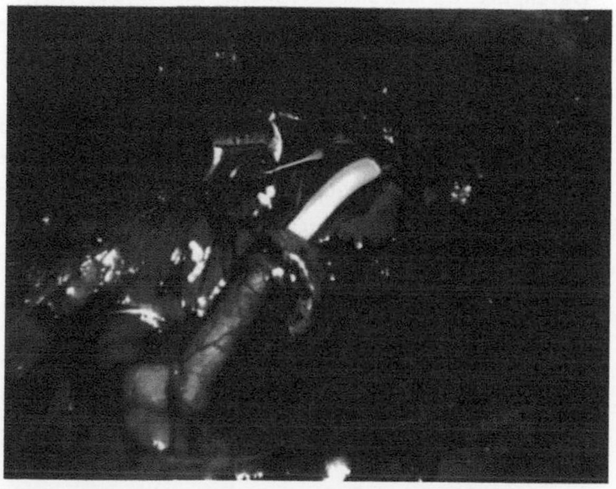

Figure 8.14 After successful stent placement, the running first suture can be started.

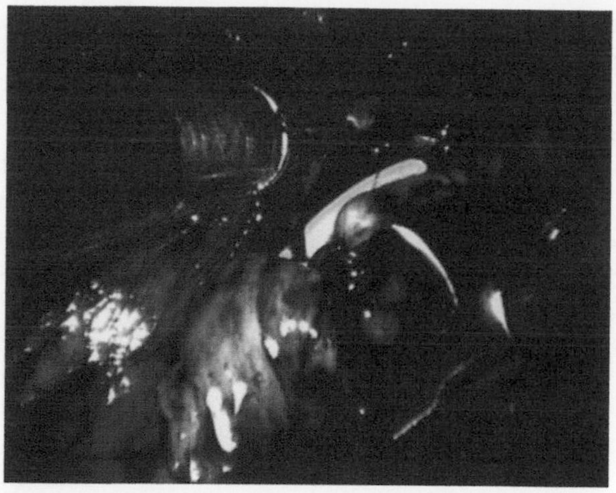

Figure 8.15 Length is an important point for the running suture. If the suture is too long, the handling may be very difficult and time-consuming. A length of 12–14 cm can be recommended.

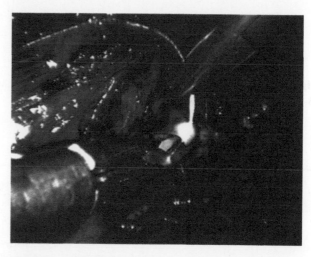

Figure 8.16 Usually, using enlargement, the stitches can be done very precisely.

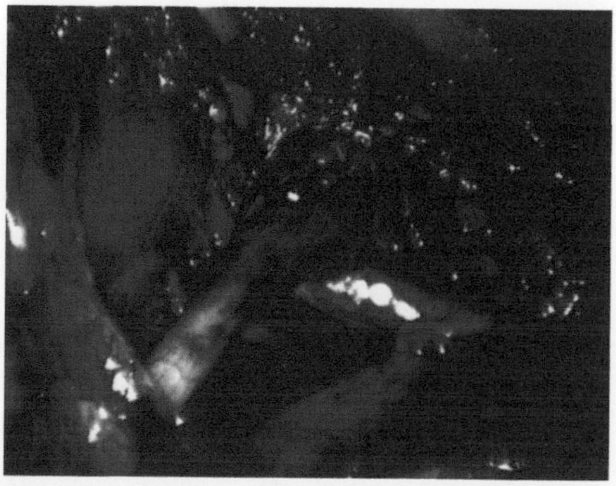

Figure 8.17 At the end, both sutures can be tied. If the renal pelvis is resected, it needs to be closed with a third suture that runs from the cranial aspect of the renal pelvis to the anastomosis.

intravenous application of a dye, which likewise leads to a sufficient demonstration of a leakage. Another method is the retrograde filling of the bladder with the dye, which can lead to a retrograde transport of the dye via the double-J stent into the renal pelvis. However, this method is less reliable. A drainage is not routinely necessary and should only be placed if a leakage cannot be completely closed. The closure of the retroperitoneum depends on the opinion of the surgeon.

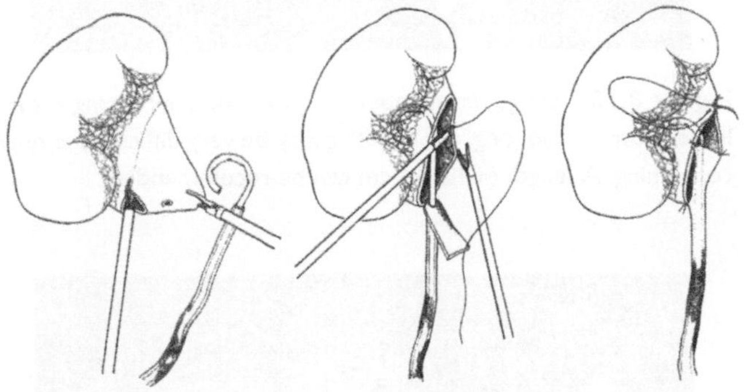

Figure 8.18 Dismembered pyeloplasty using anchor stitches (3-point fixation) to provide tension for the running sutures.

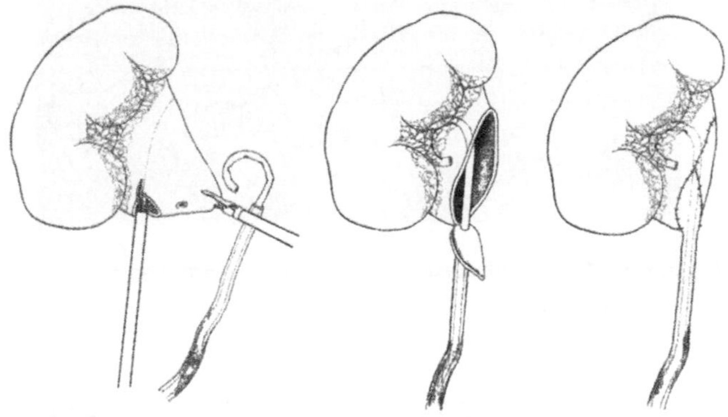

Figure 8.19 Dismembered pyeloplasty, if no renal pelvis is resected, this plasty allows the use of only two sutures.

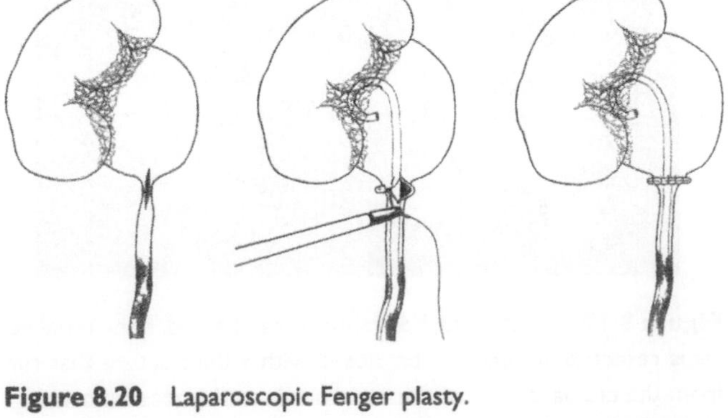

Figure 8.20 Laparoscopic Fenger plasty.

As in open surgery, there are different methods for laparoscopic pyeloplasty. The most common techniques are demonstrated in Figures 8.18–8.20.

POSTOPERATIVE SCHEDULE

- Fluid intake 2 hours after surgery
- Yoghurt 4 hours after surgery
- Mobilization on the evening of the operation day
- Diet on the first postoperative day
- Regular cost on the second postoperative day
- pain medication:
  1.5 g methamizole or 1 g paracetamol every 6 hours after surgery
  800 mg ibuprofen twice or 40 drops methamizole/paracetamol at patient's request
- Urinary catheter for 4–6 days
- Double-J stent for 4–6 weeks
- Percutaneous nephrostomy for 10 days.

REFERENCES

1. Schuessler WW, Grune MT, Tecuanhuey LV, Preminger GM. Laparoscopic dismembered pyeloplasty. J Urol 1993; 150: 1795–9.
2. Deger S, Roigas J, Wille A et al. Laparoscopic dismembered pyeloplasty with Anderson-Hynes technique. Urologe A 2003; 42: 347–53.
3. Tan HL, Roberts JP. Laparoscopic dismembered pyeloplasty in children: preliminary results. Br J Urol 1996; 77: 909–13.
4. Janetschek G, Peschel R, Bartsch G. Laparoscopic Fenger plasty. J Endourol 2000; 14: 889–93.
5. Casale P, Grady RW, Joyner BD et al. Comparison of dismembered and nondismembered laparoscopic pyeloplasty in the pediatric patient. J Endourol 2004; 18: 875–8.
6. Puppo P, Perachino M, Ricciotti G et al. Retroperitoneoscopic treatment of ureteropelvic junction obstruction. Eur Urol 1997; 31: 204–8.
7. Davenport K, Minervini A, Timoney AG, Keeley FX Jr. Our experience with retroperitoneal and transperitoneal laparoscopic pyeloplasty for pelvi-ureteric junction obstruction. Eur Urol 2005; 48: 973–7.
8. Bentas W, Wolfram M, Brautigam R et al. Da Vinci robot assisted Anderson-Hynes dismembered pyeloplasty: technique and 1 year follow-up. World J Urol 2003; 21: 133–8.
9. Olsen LH, Jorgensen TM. Computer assisted pyeloplasty in children: the retroperitoneal approach. J Urol 2004; 171: 2629–31.
10. Palese MA, Munver R, Phillips CK et al. Robot-assisted laparoscopic dismembered pyeloplasty. JSLS 2005; 9: 252–7.
11. Cascio S, Tien A, Chee W, Tan HL. Laparoscopic dismembered pyeloplasty in children younger than 2 years. J Urol 2007; 177: 335–8.
12. Metzelder ML, Schier F, Petersen C et al. Laparoscopic transabdominal pyeloplasty in children is feasible irrespective of age. J Urol 2006; 175: 688–91.

13. Sundaram CP, Grubb RL 3rd, Rehman J et al. Laparoscopic pyeloplasty for secondary ureteropelvic junction obstruction. J Urol 2003; 169: 2037–40.
14. Mandhani A, Kumar D, Kumar A et al. Steps to reduce operative time in laparoscopic dismembered pyeloplasty for moderate to large renal pelvis. Urology 2005; 66: 981–4.
15. Mandhani A, Goel S, Bhandari M. Is antegrade stenting superior to retrograde stenting in laparoscopic pyeloplasty? J Urol 2004; 171: 1440–2.
16. Romero FR, Wagner AA, Trapp C et al. Transmesenteric laparoscopic pyeloplasty. J Urol 2006; 176: 2526–9.

Part 2 Laparoscopic Surgery in the Retroperitoneal Space

CHAPTER 9

Laparoscopic retroperitoneal lymph node dissection

Andreas H Wille

INDICATIONS

The indication for laparoscopic retroperitoneal lymph node dissection (RPLND) is currently controversial, especially in stage I testicular carcinoma.[1,2] Some authors suggest primary chemotherapy (2 × PEB) as the treatment of choice in these patients to give maximum safety and avoid RLPND-related complications and morbidity. Primary RPLND does not seem to be indicated in most cases.[3]

Unfortunately the literature about laparoscopic RPLND is relatively rare, even if the published data are significant.[4–6] So, the tremendous benefits of the minimal invasive technique are not well documented compared with the considerable number of publications regarding the open technique. That is why criticism about the short term morbidity of RPLND in general is related exclusively to the open approach.

The indication for RPLND in stage II tumors or resection of residual masses after chemotherapy in stage III disease remains unaffected by the aforementioned considerations.

In our opinion laparoscopic RPLND in stage I and II disease is a worthy tool for staging with low morbidity and, besides the guidelines, we always offer the opportunity for a staging procedure to the patients if indicated.

Laparoscopic RPLND is a technically advanced procedure primarily due to the difficulty of exposure of the midline retroperitoneal structures and the presence of the great vessels with their associated branches. However, RPLND still remains the most accurate and reliable method for staging in stage I germ-cell tumors and these patients experience the usual benefits of minimally invasive surgery: less postoperative pain and narcotic use with shortened hospitalization and convalescence compared with open surgical intervention.[7]

TECHNIQUE

Basically the laparoscopic technique mimics the steps of the open modified procedure. The template for the modified laparoscopic RPLND follows that described by Donohue et al.[8] This is a modified template that is bordered, for a right-sided dissection, by the ureter laterally, the right renal vessels superiorly, the anterior surface of the aorta medially, and the inferior mesenteric artery caudally on the aorta but extending below over the inferior vena cava (IVC) and the right common iliac artery. On the left side, the borders include the left ureter laterally, the left renal vessels superiorly, and the precaval region medially. Caudally, the dissection stops at the inferior mesenteric artery over the aorta but continues lateral to the aorta and over the lateral aspect of the left common iliac artery (Figure 9.1).

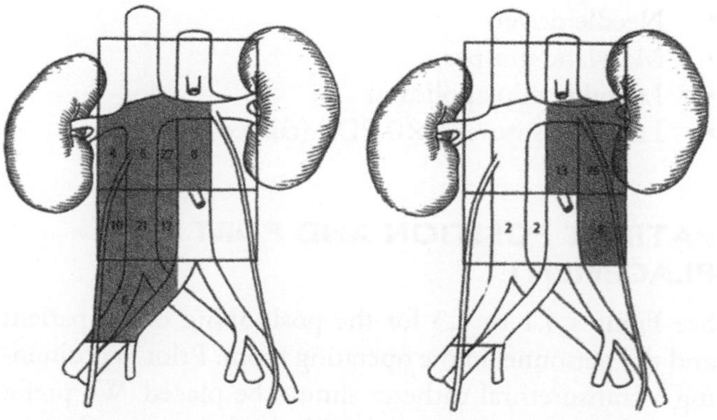

Figure 9.1 Templates for modified RPLND in stage I disease.

Surgical steps

The approach is as follows:

- mobilization of the colon
- preparation of the testicular vessels
- preparation of either the vena cava or the aorta, depending on the side of resection
- preparation of the renal vein(s)
- mobilization of the lymphatic tissue para-aortic/paracaval down to the inferior mesenteric artery
- removal of the para-aortic/paracaval tissue from the psoas muscle and the lumbal vessels
- mobilization of the interaortocaval tissue (right-sided RPLND)
- extraction of the specimen via a muscle-splitting mini incision.

PREOPERATIVE SCHEDULE

(see radical nephrectomy) in Chapter 4.

INSTRUMENTATION

- 30° optical device
- Optical port 10 mm
- Working port 5 mm (2×, optional 5 mm and 12 mm)
- Working port 10 mm
- Endo-retractor 10 mm
- Monopolar scissors
- Bipolar forceps
- Atraumatic graspers
- Clip applicator 5 mm.

Additional devices (optional)

- Stump overhold clamp 10 mm
- Endo-bulldog clamps (straight/curved)
- Clamp applicator
- Clamp remover
- Needle driver
- Maryland grasper
- Lahodny clip applicator
- Lahodny sutures 5×0 PDS (curved needle).

PATIENT POSITION AND PORT PLACEMENT

See Figures 4.1 to 4.3 for the positioning of the patient and the personnel in the operating room. Prior to positioning a transurethral catheter should be placed. We prefer the transperitoneal approach with the four-port technique as for radical nephrectomy as described earlier (Figure 9.2).

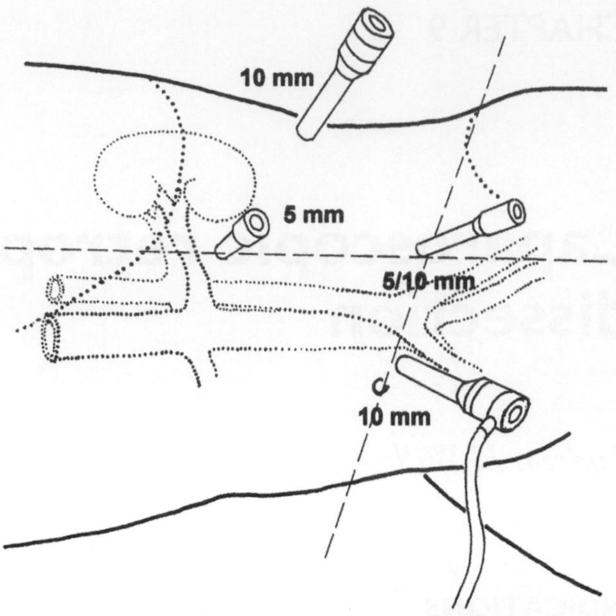

Figure 9.2 As for nephrectomy, a four-trocar technique is used.

If residual tumor resection is performed after chemotherapy the ureter may be involved in the fibrosis surrounding the tumor. In such cases a double-J stent should be inserted preoperatively. The patient is placed in the extended flank position, the camera port is inserted via an infra-umbilical incision and two additional ports are placed under direct laparoscopic vision in the mid-axillary line on either side of the first port. If standard RPLND is performed in stage I disease a 5 mm trocar can used for the lower working port if 5 mm clips (Hem-o-Lok) are available. In more difficult cases a 10 or 12 mm trocar is suggested to give the surgeon more flexibility to use the complete laparoscopic armamentarium such as large clips, suturing devices or bulldog clamps, if necessary. After mobilization of the colon a 10 mm port is inserted via a flank incision.

RIGHT-SIDED LAPAROSCOPIC RPLND

As a first step, the peritoneum is incised along the line of Toldt from the cecum to the right colic flexure. Next, the colon and the duodenum are reflected medially until the anterior wall of the aorta and the left renal vein at its crossing with the aorta are completely exposed. The testicular vein is dissected starting at the internal inguinal ring. The proximal ureter must be carefully identified because the testicular vessels pass over this structure. Special care must be taken when dissecting the junction point of the testicular vein to the inferior vena cava, since at this point the vein is liable to rupture. Avoid any traction of the testicular vein to prevent avulsion of the vena cava at the vascular junction!

The lymphatic tissue overlying the vena cava is split open, and its anterior and lateral surfaces are dissected free. Once the right and left renal veins have been dissected, the right renal artery is exposed lateral to the vena cava, and the right ureter is separated from the nodal package down to its crossing with the iliac artery. At this point, the lymph node package is clipped and transected. Next, the lymphatic tissue overlying the common iliac artery and the aorta is split from caudal in an ascending direction. As the dissection is continued cephalad, care must be taken to preserve the inferior mesenteric artery. Cranially to the artery, the lymphatic tissue is split along the left border of the aorta so that the ventral surface of the aorta is completely freed. Now the right renal artery can be identified as it courses across the interaortocaval space, and the upper border of the dissection becomes well delineated. The dissection then continues into the interaortocaval region. This dissection must proceed very cautiously due to the variability of the network of small vascular branches off the great vessels. The dissection is carried down to the lumbar vessels, and the interaortocaval package is removed step by step. As a last step, the nodal package on the right side of the vena cava is removed. The specimen is harvested with an endo-bag using the lateral port incision.

LEFT-SIDED LAPAROSCOPIC RPLND

The access is established as described above for the right side and the procedure is performed in a similar way, although template size and localization are different. The boundaries of the template are the left ureter laterally, the renal vessels superiorly, and include all tissue lateral to the aorta and the preaortic tissue cranial to the inferior mesenteric artery. The interaortocaval nodes are not removed. Again, the line of Toldt is incised and the descending colon is mobilized to expose the aorta and the iliac artery. Mobilization of the spleen is necessary in most cases to ensure optimal access. Now the anterior surface of the aorta is completely exposed. The testicular vein is removed and the left renal vein is freed completely. Care should be taken when resecting the lumbar vein that usually enters the renal vein at its dorsal aspect. Subsequently, the nodal package is removed using the same technique as for the right side. The dissection is carried down to the level of the lumbar arteries without resecting them. Watch out for the thoracic duct, which can be damaged during this maneuver causing significant chylous ascites postoperatively! Always use clips for large lymphatic vessels!

RESECTION OF RESIDUAL MASSES AFTER CHEMOTHERAPY IN HIGHER STAGE DISEASE

The principles and techniques are basically the same as described above. The high amount of fibrotic tissue usually present after chemotherapy is challenging to the surgeon's skills. Caval adhesions are difficult to handle, particularly if the junction of the testicular vein is involved. Traction of the adherent tissue may cause unexpected major bleeding due to damage of large vessels. The indication has to be very careful and a primary open approach should be considered.

LAPARSCOPIC RPLND STEP BY STEP

Staging procedure in left-sided non-seminomatous germ-cell tumor (stage I disease)

The procedure is illustrated in Figures 9.3–9.6.

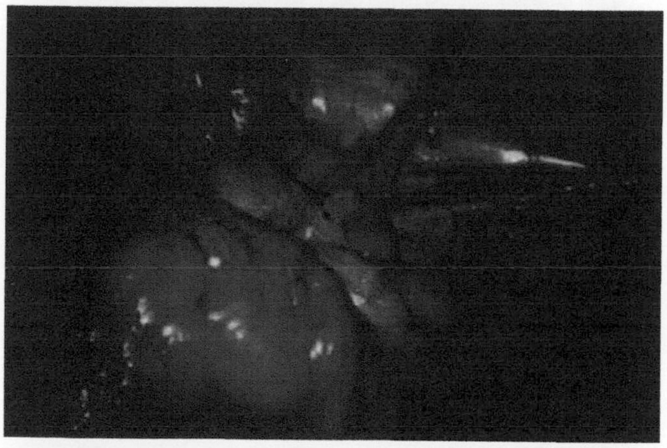

Figure 9.3 Mobilization of the colon descendens. The testicular vessels are exposed.

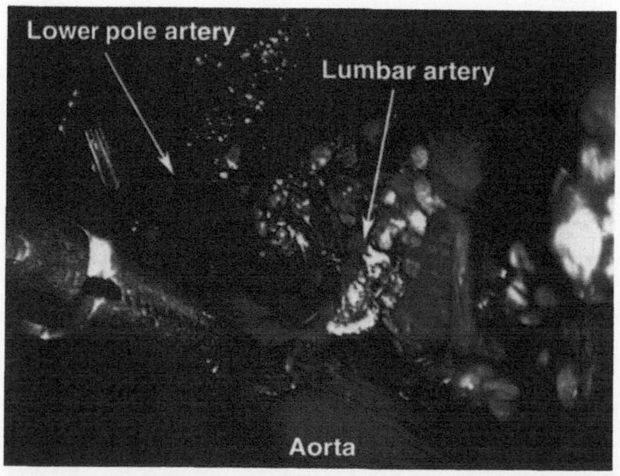

Figure 9.4 Preparation of the hilar tissue. The aorta is completely free and the proximal ureter is saved. A lower pole artery and a lumbar artery are visualized and spared.

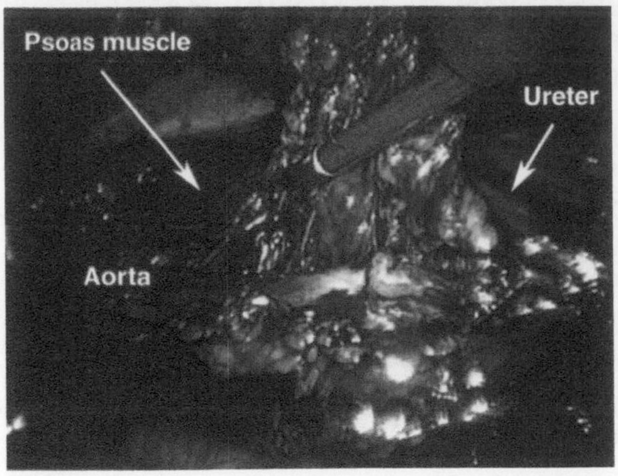

Figure 9.5 Distal portion of the template. The lymphatic tissue between the ureter and the cranial part of the iliac artery has been mobilized.

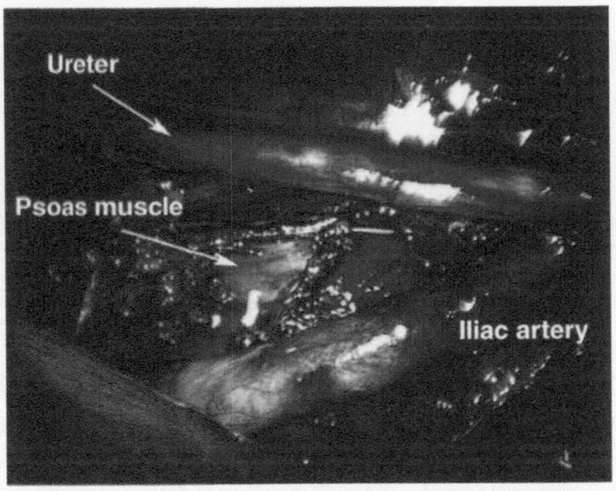

Figure 9.6 Lymphatic tissue has been removed. The aorta, iliac artery, and ureter are mobilized, the psoas muscle is visible.

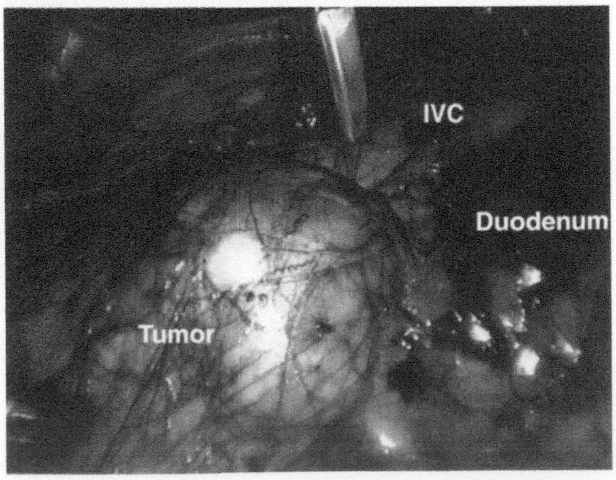

Figure 9.7 Interaortocaval tumor mass adherent to the vena cava. The duodenum is attached.

Single interaortocaval lymph node metastasis in right non-seminomatous germ-cell tumor (stage II disease), right-sided access

This procedure is illustrated in Figures 9.7–9.11.

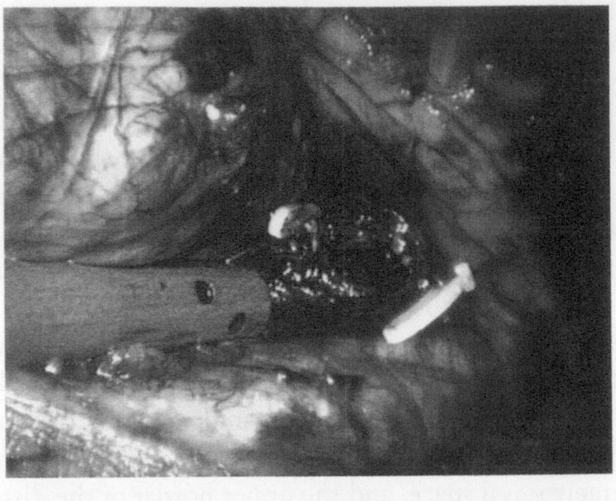

Figure 9.8 The duodenum has been mobilized and lymphatic strands are clipped with 5 mm Hem-o-Lok clips.

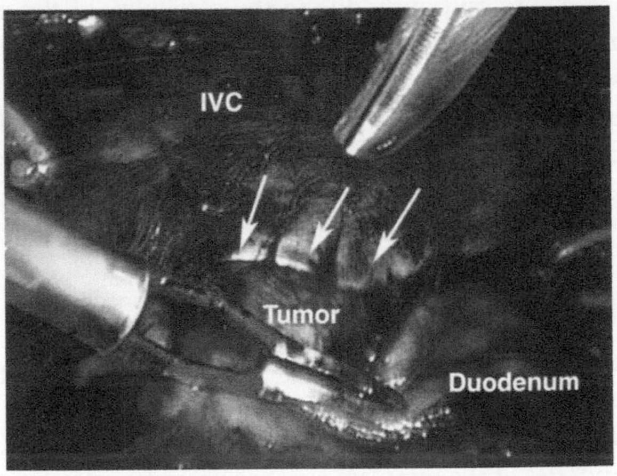

Figure 9.9 Adhesions between the tumor and left wall of the vena cava are carefully resected.

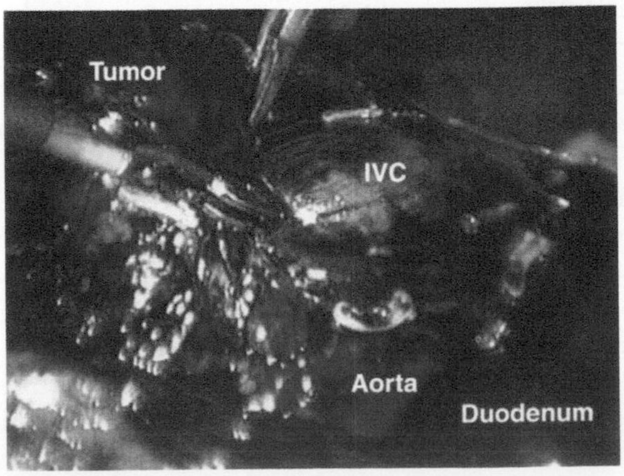

Figure 9.10 The tumor is moved laterally and the main lymph tissue is exposed for resection.

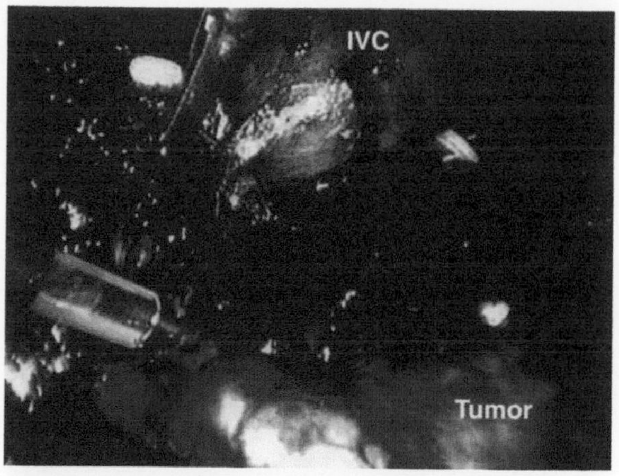

Figure 9.11 The tumor is moved medially to complete mobilization off the vena cava and the dorsal aspect.

POSTOPERATIVE SCHEDULE

See nephrectomy in Chapter 4.

REFERENCES

1. Weissbach L, Bussar-Maatz R, Flechtner H et al. RPLND or primary chemotherapy in clinical stage IIA/B nonseminomatous germ cell tumors? Results of a prospective multicenter trial including quality of life assessment. Eur Urol 2000; 37: 582–94.
2. Yoon GH, Stein JP, Skinner DG. Retroperitoneal lymph node dissection in the treatment of low-stage nonseminomatous germ cell tumors of the testicle: an update. Urol Oncol 2005; 23: 168–77.
3. Albers P. Management of stage I testis cancer. Eur Urol 2007; 51(1): 34–43.
4. Abdel-Aziz KF, Anderson JK, Svatek R et al. Laparoscopic and open retroperitoneal lymph-node dissection for clinical stage I nonseminomatous germ cell testis tumors. J Endourol 2006; 20: 627–31.
5. Steiner H, Peschel R, Janetschek G et al. Long term results of laparoscopic retroperitoneal lymph node dissection: a single center 10-year experience. Urology 2004; 63: 550–5.
6. Albqami N, Janetschek G. Laparoscopic retroperitoneal lymph-node dissection in the management of clinical stage I and II testicular cancer. J Endourol 2005; 19: 683–92.
7. Poulakis V, Skriapas K, de Vries R et al. Quality of life after laparoscopic and open retroperitoneal lymph node dissection in clinical stage I nonseminomatous germ cell tumors: a comparison study. Urology 2006; 68: 154–60.
8. Donohue JP, Foster RS, Rowland RG et al. Nerve-sparing retroperitoneal lymphadenectomy with preservation of ejaculation. J Urol 1990; 144: 287–91; discussion 291–2.

CHAPTER 10

Laparoscopic fenestration of renal cysts

Markus Giessing

INDICATION

The incidence of renal cysts is about 50% of the adult population, and the increase of distribution of imaging techniques (sonography, CT) has led to an increase in their detection. Simple renal cysts occur in about 20% of the population at 40 years and 33% at 60 years. In rare cases renal cysts may be associated with renal tumors (M. Hippel Lindau, tuberous sclerosis).[1,2]

Based on CT scan renal cysts are classified in four categories according to Bosniak[3] (Table 10.1).

Treatment indications are as follows:

- Bosniak I/II: flank pain, hypertension, hematuria, infection, obstruction of collecting system
- Bosniak III/IV: treatment always indicated
- Peripelvic cysts Urinary outflow obstruction

Treatment of Bosniak I cysts can be performed by percutaneous aspiration with or without injection of sclerosants, open marsupialization, open surgery, or by laparoscopic (transperitoneal or retroperitoneal) approach. The surgical approach renders the best results. Laparoscopy is the least invasive therapy for optimal treatment. Bosniak II cysts can be treated laparoscopically with intraoperative cyst aspiration and biopsies, followed by (partial) nephrectomy in case of malignancy.[4] Bosniak III/IV cysts should be treated by removal of the cyst or (partial) nephrectomy. Laparoscopy is the least invasive surgical option. Laparoscopic cyst aspiration and biopsies for Bosniak III cysts, followed by (partial) nephrectomy in case of malignancy has also been described.[4] Peripelvic cysts can be handled by laparoscopy as well. Experience is limited as yet, as only about 50 cases have been reported in the literature.[5] Operative strategy for peripelvic cysts differs from the strategy described below in placing an open-ended ureteral stent before the operation in order to be able to install a dye (methylene blue/indigo carmine) intraoperatively to exclude accidental injury of the renal pelvis.[1,2,5]

PREOPERATIVE SCHEDULE

- CT for Bosniak classification and localization
- Enema administered at 18:00/20:00
- Anticoagulation s.c. at 20:00
- Cleaning of umbilicus.

INSTRUMENTATION

A laparoscopy set is required, as in (partial) nephrectomy:

- trocars: two 10 mm and two 5 mm
- laparoscopy coagulation device (bipolar is best)
- laparoscopy graspers, scissors
- laparoscopy aspiration needle
- laparoscopy suction device
- laparoscopy needle holder
- (laparoscopy specimen retrieval bag)

Table 10.1 Imaging features in CT of renal cysts according to Bosniak classification

Bosniak class	*Imaging features*
I	Simple cyst, no enhancement after injection of contrast medium, < 20 (−50) Houndsfield units ⇒ benign
II	Homogenous hyperdense cyst, thin septs/fine calcification, no enhancement after injection of contrast medium ⇒ mostly benign
III	Multiloculated cystic mass or cyst with thick irregular calcifications/thick wall or nodularity, enhancement after injection of contrast medium ⇒ mostly malignant
IV	Cyst associated with solid component, enhancement after injection of contrast medium ⇒ mostly malignant

Optional: equipment may be required for preoperative ureteral stenting (this should always be performed in peripelvic cysts).

STEP-BY-STEP OPERATIVE TECHNIQUE

- Four-trocar transperitoneal technique (in analogy to nephrectomy trocar sites)
- Optional preoperative ureteral stenting.

Trocars are removed under vision to exclude incisional bleedings. For trocars larger than 10 mm the fascia should be sutured under visual control. Complete desufflation at the end of the operation is important to prevent abdominal and shoulder pain. Subcutaneous suture is optional. Skin closure should be performed with intracutaneous rapidly resorbable sutures.

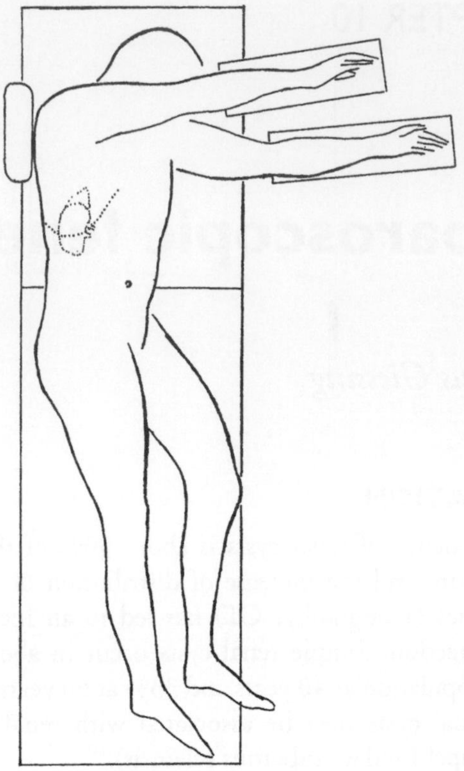

Figure 10.2 The position of the patient on the operation table. The patient is in lumbar position, flexed between the inferior costal margin and the spina iliaca anterior superior. The lower arm is extended (be careful with the shoulder) and the upper arm is angled.

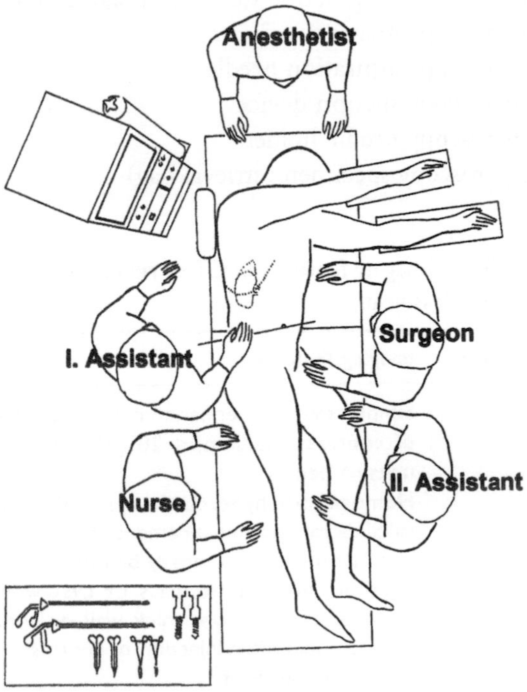

Figure 10.1 Positions of the patient, surgeon and nurse in the operation room. The surgeon is on the ventral side of the patient, cephalad of the assistant; the assistant is on the ventral side of the patient for the camera; the nurse is on the dorsal side of the patient.

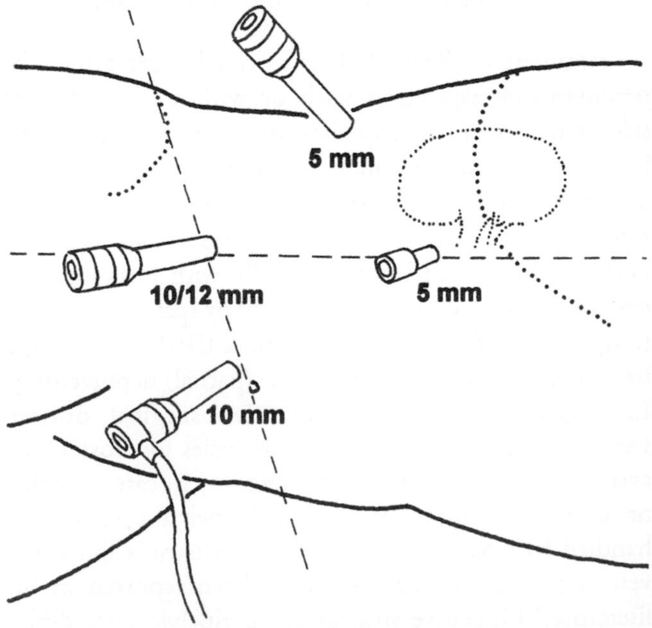

Figure 10.3 The position of the trocars for the operation field. Four-trocar technique: 10 mm optical trocar infra-umbilical, 5 mm trocar in medioclavicular line subcostally, 10 mm trocar in medioclavicular line a little below the optical trocar.

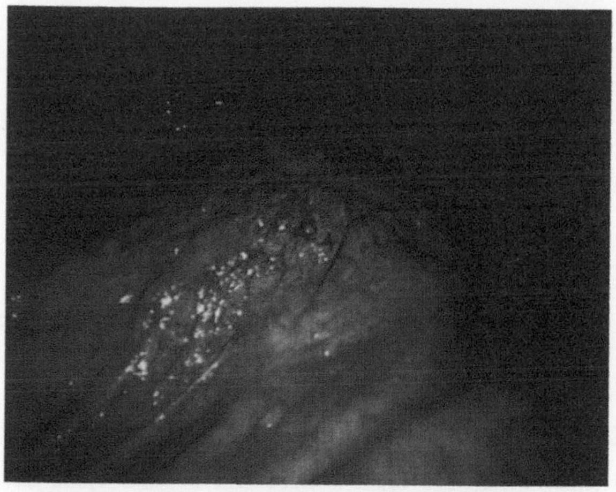

Figure 10.4 Identification of renal cyst. Ventral and lateral cysts may be visible without mobilizing the colon, nevertheless, the colon has to be dissected carefully.

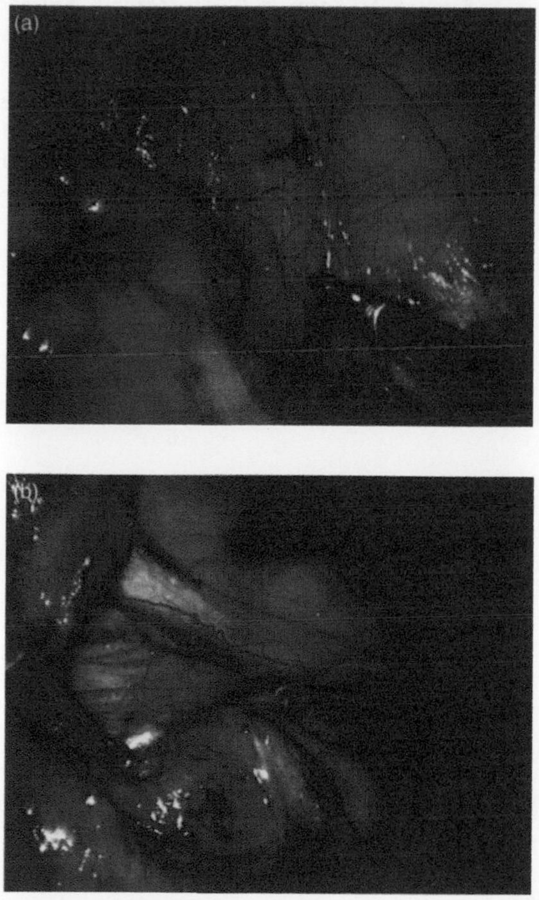

Figure 10.5 (a) Mobilizing the upper colon. For access to the kidney cyst, depending on its localization, the colon ascendens (for the left side) or descendens (right side) has to be mobilized as in laparoscopic nephrectomy along the Toldt line. (b) Mobilizing the lower colon. Usually, for best visibility and control, the lower part of the colon should also be mobilized. This is especially indicated for dorsal cysts, as the kidney itself may have to be pulled ventrally and adherent colon can be in the way. The right plane is indicated by visualization of the ureter, the gonadal vein, and the psoas muscle.

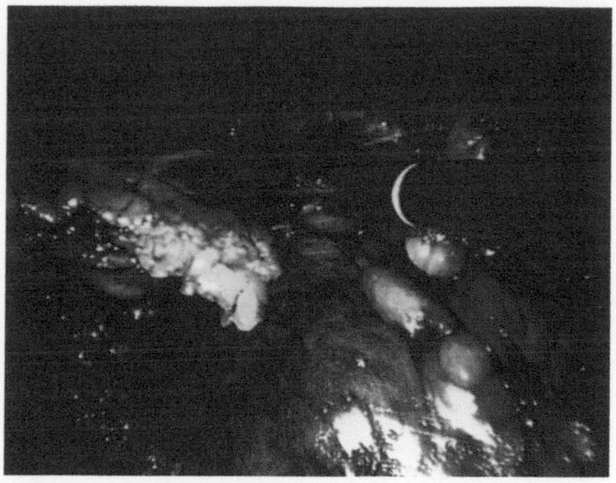

Figure 10.6 Complete visualization of the cyst. The renal cyst is visualized completely by dissecting adherent fatty tissue. This step has to be carried out very carefully, as the wall of the cyst may be very thin.

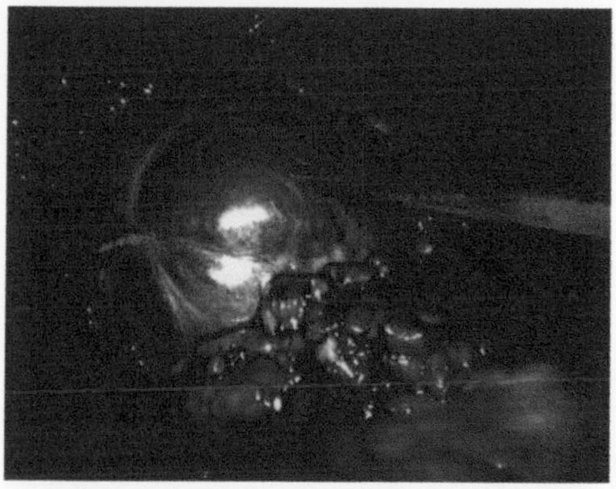

Figure 10.7 Aspiration of the cyst. If the strategy of the operation depends on the result of fluid aspiration, this should be performed before extensive dissection. The whole of the aspiration needle can be sutured to prevent fluid spilling. If intraoperative histology reveals a malignant cyst, nephrectomy or partial nephrectomy can be performed laparoscopically.

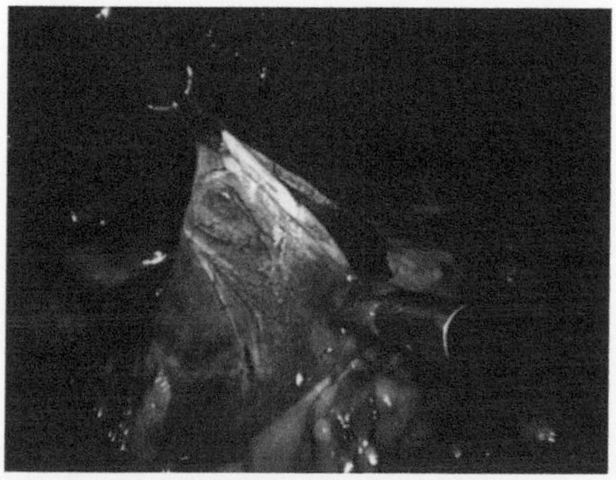

Figure 10.8 Incision of the cyst wall. In case of a Bosniak I cyst or negative findings for fluid aspiration of a Bosniak II (III) cyst the wall is incised with graspers and a pair of scissors.

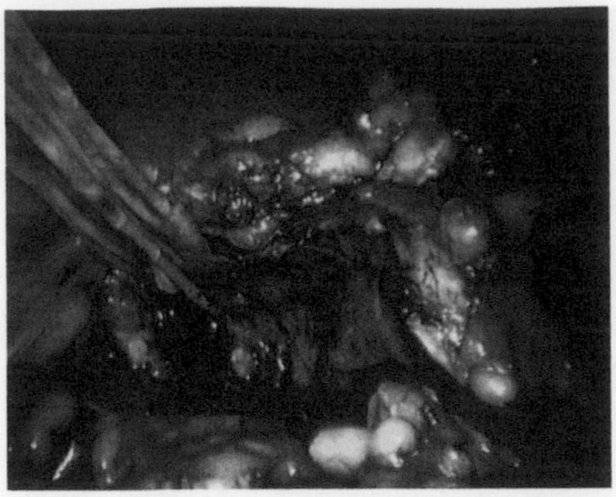

Figure 10.9 Circumferential excision of cyst wall, coagulation, biopsies. The complete wall of the cyst is removed. Bipolar coagulation of the rim prevents it from bleeding. Biopsies can now be taken from the cyst material or from suspicious areas. They should be sent for frozen section, so as to be able to continue with the operation (partial or total nephrectomy) in case of malignancy.

POSTOPERATIVE SCHEDULE

- Operation day
  mobilization 4–6 hours after operation
  urinary output control
  yoghurt and tea (time according to anesthesiologist)/add infusions
  thrombosis prophylaxis
  pain medication
- Postoperative day 1
  ultrasound
  serum creatinine
  light diet/no further infusion
  complete mobilization
  thrombosis prophylaxis
  pain medication
- Postoperative day 2
  discharge (when no complications have occurred).

REFERENCES

1. Hemal AK. Laparoscopic management of renal cystic disease. Urol Clin North Am 2001; 28: 115–26.
2. Kreft B, Schild HH. Cystical renal lesions. Fortschr Röntgenstr 2003; 175: 892–903.
3. Bosniak MA. The current radiological approach to renal cysts. Radiology 1986; 158: 1–10.
4. Limb J, Santiago L, Kaswick J. Laparoscopic evaluation of indeterminate renal cysts: long-term follow-up. J Endourol 2002; 16: 79–82.
5. Camargo AH, Cooperberg MR, Ershoff BD et al. Laparoscopic management of peripelvic renal cysts: University of California, San Francisco, experience and review of the literature. Urology 2005; 65: 882–7.

CHAPTER 11

Laparoscopic pelvic lymph adenectomy

Jan Roigas

INDICATION

Laparoscopic lymph node dissection is a common surgical procedure. It was described at the beginning of the 1990s using the transperitoneal laparoscopic and also the retroperitoneal approach.[1,2] In most cases, this operation will be performed as a staging procedure in patients with prostate cancer, either during radical laparoscopic prostatectomy or prior to perineal prostatectomy, or as a staging procedure before the different forms of radiation therapy.

In rare cases, this procedure provides a diagnostic or prognostic tool for penile cancer or for muscle invasive bladder cancer before or during radical cystectomy.

Laparoscopic lymph node dissection can be performed as a staging or an extended procedure; the staging procedure is more common. This operation provides an excellent learning opportunity for the novice laparoscopic surgeon, while the extended approach requires advanced laparoscopic skills. However, in experienced centers the extended approach does not seem to be associated with a higher morbidity for the patient.[3]

For prostate cancer the indication for laparoscopic lymph node dissection has changed over recent years. Currently, there is great acceptance to perform this diagnostic operation only in high-risk patients (as defined by a PSA >10 ng/ml, a Gleason sum > 7 or on the basis of nomograms). Laparoscopic lymph node staging seems to be more accurate than MRI or CT for these high-risk patients.[4] Modern approaches, based on the sentinel node concept, use laparoscopy for the extraction of radio-labeled sentinel nodes, which may be located outside the common standard lymphadenectomy area.[5]

Beside these experimental approaches for lymph node staging in prostate cancer, classical staging lymphadenectomy remains a standard tool in the staging of high-risk prostate cancer patients in particular.

PREOPERATIVE SCHEDULE

- Diet: Patients can have a normal breakfast in the morning, soup for lunch, and fluid only in the evening.
- Bowel preparation: No specific bowel preparation is necessary. Two rectal enemas are administered in the evening.
- Perioperative antibiotic treatment: Third-generation cephalosporin is used as a single shot during surgery.

INSTRUMENTATION

- 2 trocars (10 mm)
- 2 trocars (5 mm)
- Optical system (10 mm, 0°) for second assistant
- Scissors for surgeon
- Grasper or bipolar grasper (optional) for surgeon
- Suction device for first assistant.

POSITIONING OF THE PATIENT/ OPERATIVE TECHNIQUE

The patient is positioned in the operating room on his back in a 10–20° Trendelenburg position (Figures 11.1 and 11.2). A catheter has to be placed into the bladder to avoid bladder injury during trocar placement.

Following infra-umbilical incision, placement of the Veress needle, and establishment of the pneumoperitoneum, four trocars have to be placed. As well as the 10 mm optical trocar at the infra-umbilical site, two 5 mm trocars have to be placed under visual control in the pararectal region in the middle of the line between the umbilicus and spina iliaca anterior superior. It is strongly recommended that these trocars are not placed in a very caudal position, since this will hinder the access to the fossa obturatoria.

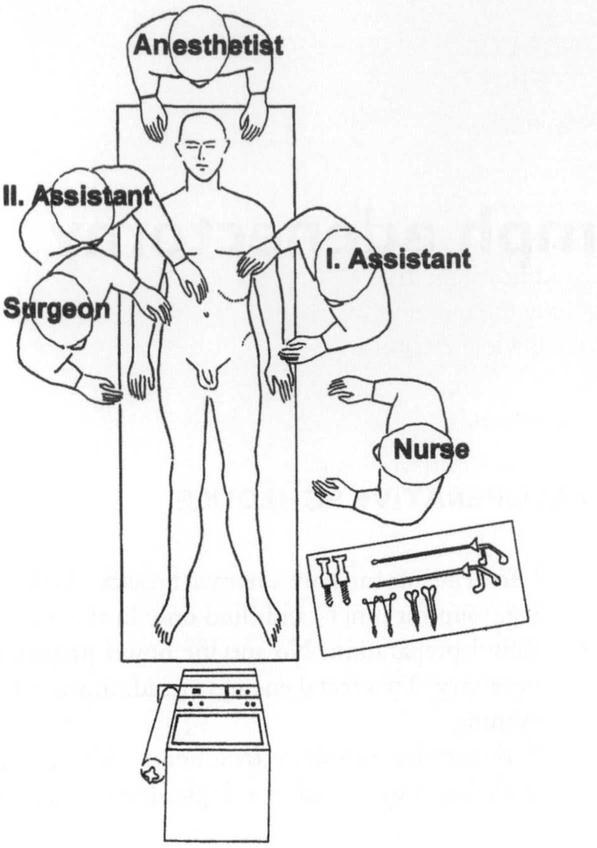

Figure 11.1 Scheme of the organization in the operating room.

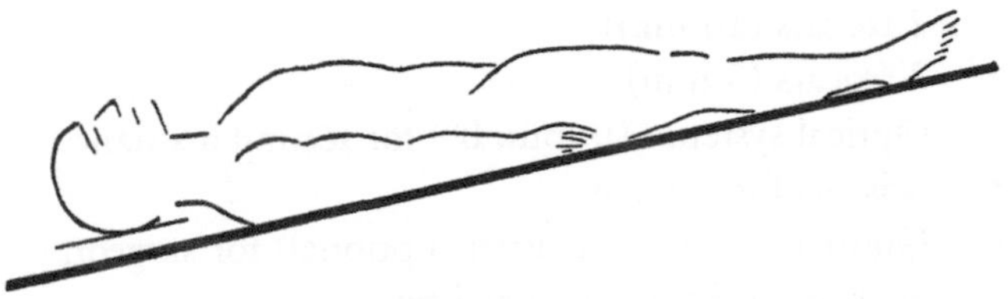

Figure 11.2 The patient is positioned in a 10–20° Trendelenburg position.

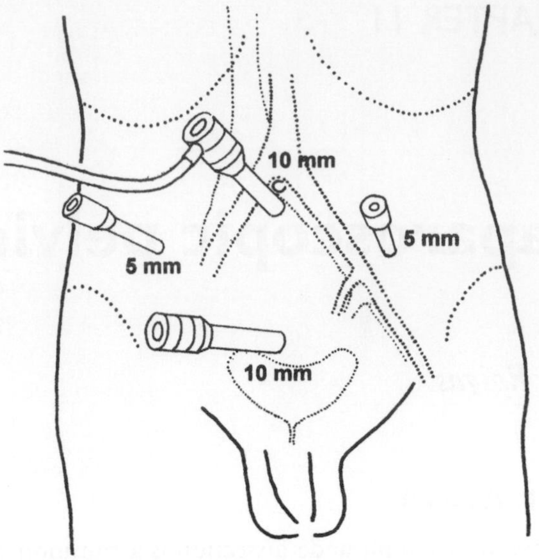

Figure 11.3 The placmenent of the four trocars is as follows: one 10 mm optical trocar infra-umbilical, two 5 mm trocars pararectal in the middle of the line between the umbilicus and spina iliaca anterior superior, one 10 mm trocar in the midline directly above the bladder dome.

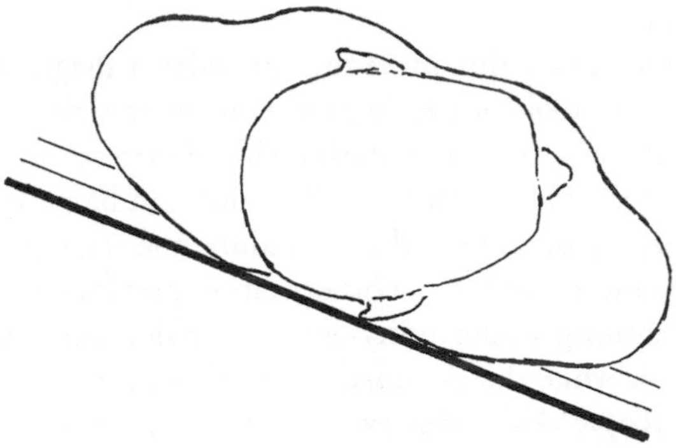

Figure 11.4 The patient is lifted up on the operating side.

The fourth trocar needs to be placed in the midline directly above the bladder dome between the two plicae (Figure 11.3). Assistance with a 5 mm grasper is very useful for the placement of this 10 mm trocar. In difficult cases urine should be controlled. The occurrence of sanguineous urine may be a sign of a bladder injury.

After all trocars have been placed the peritoneal cavity should be inspected. Then the patient should be lifted up on the operation side and the view should be focused on the operating field (Figure 11.4). Figures 11.5 and 11.6 demonstrate important anatomic landmarks, such as the external iliac vessels, the ureter, the internal inguinal ring with the testicular vessels, the ductus deferens, and the plicae umbilicales laterales.

The surgical procedure should start with the long incision of the peritoneum directly above the external iliac artery (Figure 11.7). The long incision is important to avoid the formation of lymphoceles in the postoperative phase. In obese patients it may be difficult to identify the external iliac artery. In these cases, it is recommended that the peritoneum is observed for detection of a progagated arterial pulsing. It is useful to keep anatomic landmarks in mind to avoid the preparation of the internal iliac artery. If the external iliac artery cannot be securely identified, then the incision of the peritoneum medially from the testicular vessels is advised.

Following the preparation of the artery (Figure 11.8) the identification of the external iliac vein is the next surgical step. Usually, by pulling the median margin of the incised peritoneum medially, the lateral margin of the vein can be seen. With blunt preparations using the scissors, the vein can be separated from surrounding tissue. The medial margin of the vein is the anatomic landmark at that point (Figure 11.9).

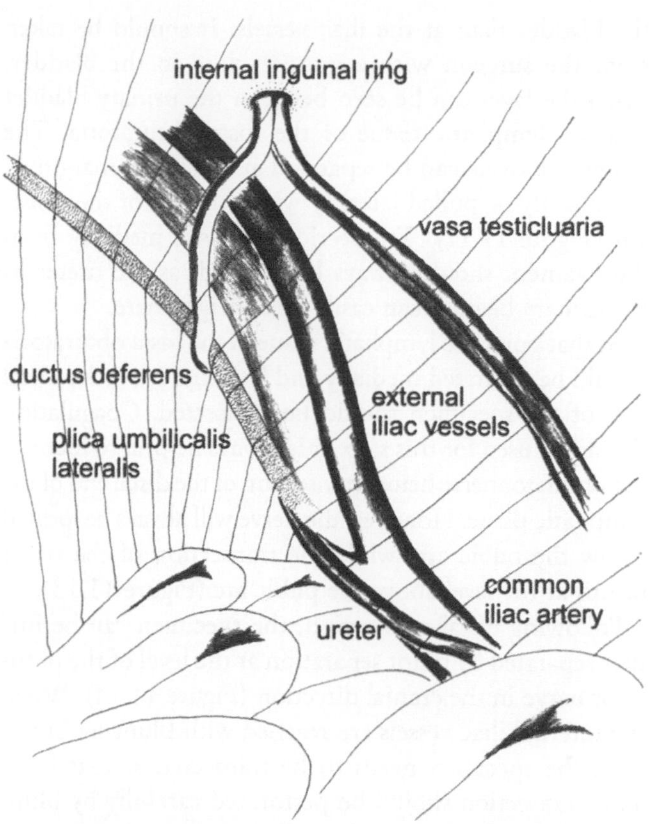

Figure 11.5 Important anatomic structures are: external iliac vessels, plica umbilicalis lateralis, testicular vessels, ductus deferens, and ureter.

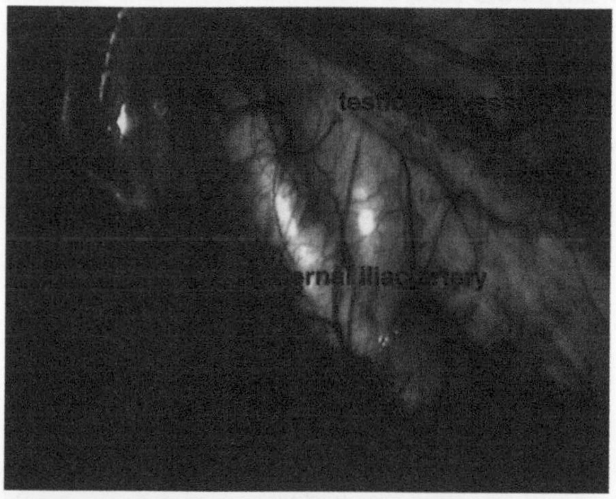

Figure 11.6 Anatomic landmarks should be identified before incision of the peritoneum.

The incision of the peritoneum up to the ductus deferens should be performed distally. The ductus deferens can be transected by carefully controlling the arteria ductus deferentis for bleeding. For the novice surgeon the transection of the ductus deferens alleviates the further separation of the lymphatic tissue. However, the ductus deferens can also be kept intact, but should then be separated in the direction of the urinary bladder.

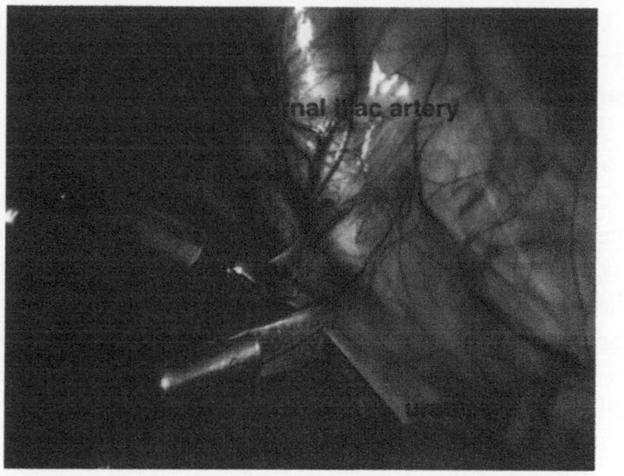

Figure 11.7 Incision of the parietal peritoneum above the external iliac artery using a bipolar grasper and monopolar scissors. Monopolar coagulation should only be used very carefully.

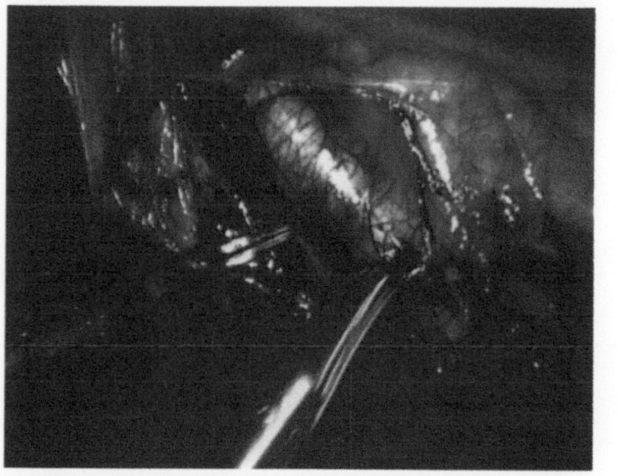

Figure 11.8 The incision of the peritoneum and preparation of the external iliac artery should be long enough to avoid the formation of lymphoceles.

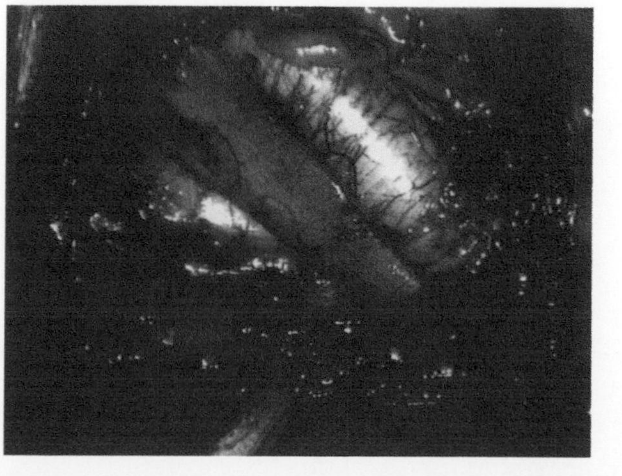

Figure 11.9 When the external iliac vein is separated, the preparation of the lateral aspect of the lymphatic tissue can be performed directly from its medial margin.

Cranially, the peritoneal incision has to be performed very carefully to avoid injuries to the ureter and the internal iliac artery.

The next step is the separation of the lymphatic tissue from the medial margin of the external iliac vein and the identification of the musculus obturatorius internus and the pubic bone (Figure 11.10). It is very helpful if the assistant carefully pulls the vein laterally with a grasper or the suction device. At the musculature, the lymphatic tissue can be easily pulled down with the scissors. Blood vessels for the musculature should be coagulated and transected (Figure 11.11).

Following this lateral preparation the identification of the plica umbilicalis lateralis is the next step. Sometimes, especially in obese patients, it is difficult to identify the ligamentum umbilicale laterale (or chorda arteriae umbilicalis). The ligament can be found more easily at the bladder than at the iliac vessels. It should be taken from the surgeon with a grasper close to the bladder. Then the layer can be seen between the urinary bladder and the lymphatic tissue of the fossa obturatoria. The lymphatic tissue can be separated at its medial margin. It can bluntly be pulled laterally with the help of the assistant (Figure 11.12). Transection of tissue medially from the ligament should always be avoided, as the ureter or the urinary bladder can easily be damaged here.

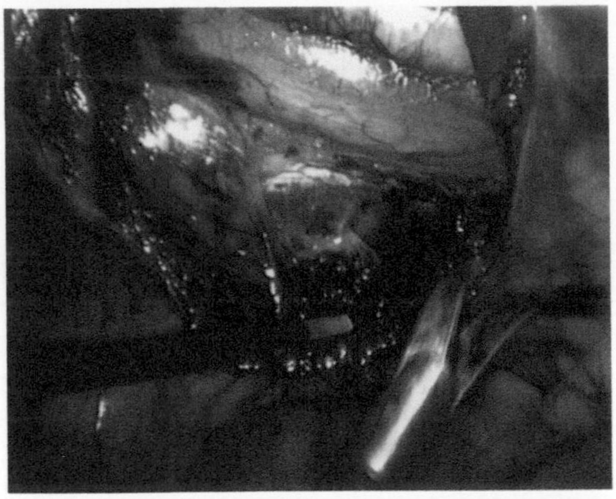

Figure 11.10 The identification of the musculus obturatorius internus and the pubic arc is important. These structures represent the lateral border of the operation field.

At that point the lymphatic tissue of the fossa obturatoria should be separated medially and laterally. Now the distal end of the specimen should be transected. Coagulation should be used for this step. It is always helpful to identify the obturator nerve before transection of the distal end of the lymphatic tissue. However, the nerve will always be located below the pubic arc, while the transection of the tissue begins at the level above the pubic arc (Figure 11.13).

Following distal transection, the specimen can be further separated by blunt separation at the level of the obturator nerve in the cranial direction (Figure 11.14). When the internal iliac vessels are reached with blunt mobilization, the specimen needs to be transected at that level. This transection should be performed carefully by blunt and sharp tissue separation (Figure 11.15). Attention needs to be paid to the obturator nerve, the oburator artery, and the internal vessels, especially the internal iliac vein. In most cases the ureter is located more cranially and medially of this area, and therefore it is not an anatomical structure that can easily be damaged during lymphatic tissue transection.

When the lymphatic tissue is completely separated it should be carefully removed from the peritoneal space, either by

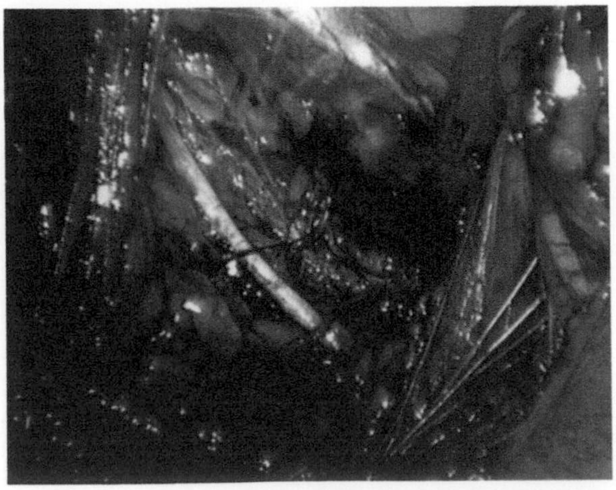

Figure 11.11 In the deep, the nervus obturatorius and the obturator vessels can be identified. In a simple staging procedure, no further and deeper preparation is required.

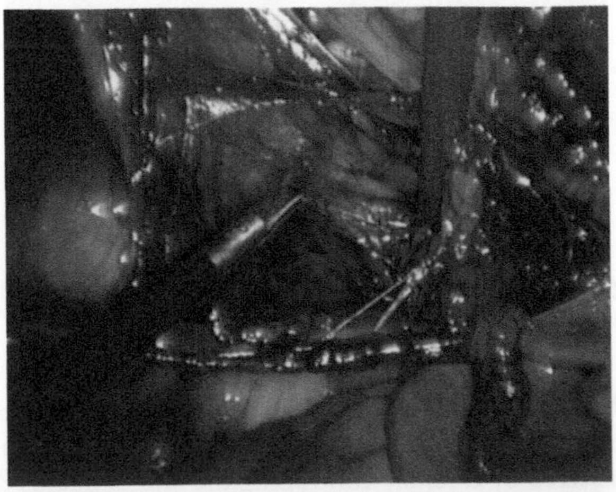

Figure 11.12 If the ligamentum umbilicale laterale is taken with the surgeon's grasper, the layer between urinary bladder and the lymphatic tissue can be identified and the assistant can pull the specimen laterally. The specimen can be mobilized with blunt and sharp preparation with the scissors.

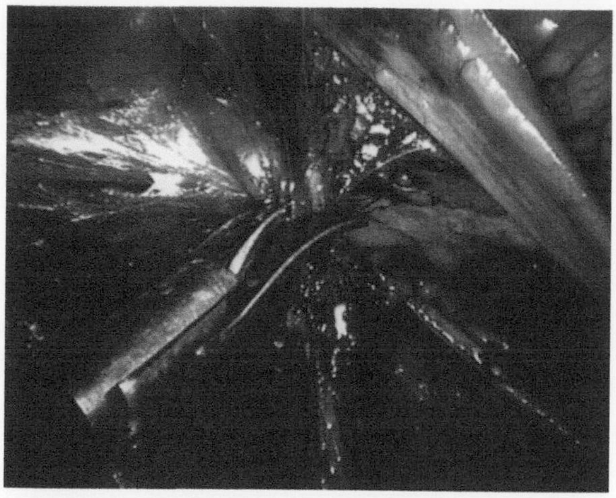

Figure 11.13 The distal aspect of the specimen is transected.

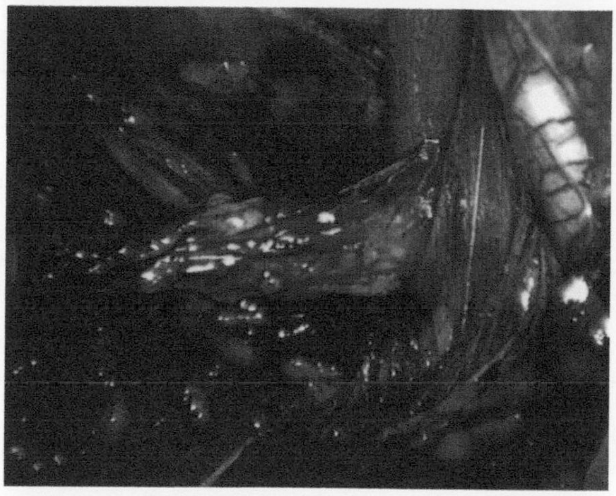

Figure 11.14 With blunt mobilization the lymphatic tissue can be separated at the cranial aspect of the operating field.

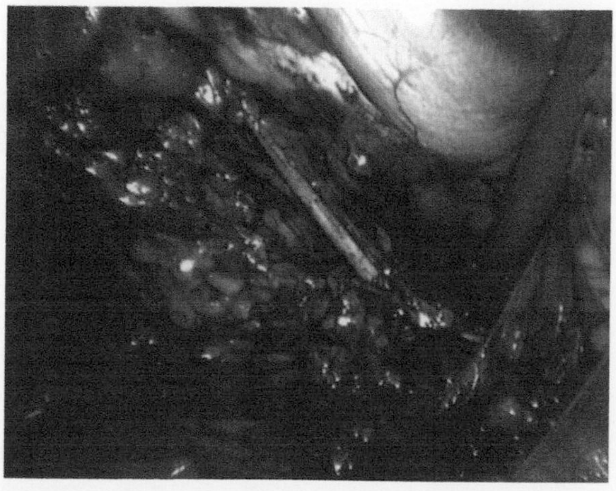

Figure 11.15 During the transection of the tissue attention has to be paid to the internal iliac vessels and the obturator nerve.

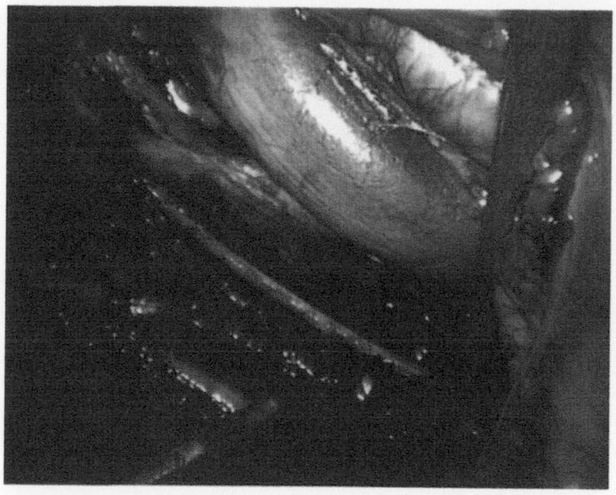

Figure 11.16 Final view of the operating field demonstrating the obturator nerve, the obturator vessels, the ligamentum umbilicalis lateralis, and the external iliac vessels.

using an endo-bag or with a large grasper under visual control. Finally the operating field should be inspected carefully for bleedings or lesions of adjacent organs (Figure 11.16). It is not necessary to place a drainage routinely.

POSTOPERATIVE SCHEDULE

- Fluid intake 2 hours after surgery
- Yoghurt 4 hours after surgery
- Mobilization on the evening of the operation day
- Diet on the first postoperative day
- Regular cost on the second postoperative day.
- pain medication:

  1.5 g methamizole or 1 g paracetamol every 6 hours after surgery
  800 mg ibuprofen twice or 40 drops methamizole/ paracetamol at the patient's request.

REFERENCES

1. Schuessler WW, Vancaillie TG, Reich H, Griffith DP. Transperitoneal endosurgical lymphadenectomy in patients with localized prostate cancer. J Urol 1991; 145: 988–91.
2. Ferzli G, Trapasso J, Raboy A, Albert P. Extraperitoneal endoscopic pelvic lymph node dissection. J Laparoendosc Surg 1992; 2: 39–44.
3. Wyler SF, Sulser T, Seifert HH et al. Laparoscopic extended pelvic lymph node dissection for high-risk prostate cancer. Urology 2006; 68: 883–7.
4. Borley N, Fabrin K, Sriprasad S et al. Laparoscopic pelvic lymph node dissection allows significantly more accurate staging in "high-risk" prostate cancer compared to MRI or CT. Scand J Urol Nephrol 2003; 37: 382–6.
5. Corvin S, Schilling D, Eichhorn K et al. Laparoscopic sentinel lymph node dissection – a novel technique for the staging of prostate cancer. Eur Urol 2006; 49: 280–5.

CHAPTER 12

Laparoscopic adrenalectomy – transperitoneal approach

Mario Zacharias

INDICATION

The transperitoneal approach to laparoscopic adrenalectomy is indicated for the removal of non-functional and functional solid adrenal masses of small to intermediate size. This includes masses of the adrenal cortex – aldosteromas, glucocorticoid-, androgen-, and estrogen-producing adenomas, solitary small pheochromocytomas, hormone-inactive lesions larger than 3 cm that demonstrate growth over time on serial imaging studies, tumours larger than 4–5 cm without observation, adrenal cysts or myelolipomas, and selected cases of bilateral adrenal hyperplasia.

Special indications are the removal of malignant tumors or metastases. The criteria for performing laparoscopic surgery on these tumors include controllability of the primary cancer, resectability of any other metastatic lesion, and physical fitness of the patient to tolerate general anesthesia.

PREOPERATIVE SCHEDULE

General recommendations

- A mechanical bowel preparation is not necessary.
- Thrombosis prevention (low-molecular-weight heparin) is mandatory.
- Single-shot intravenous antibiosis using a cephalosporin should be administered at the beginning of the procedure.

Pharmacological management in pheochromocytoma patients

- The preoperative medical treatment of choice is the long-acting alpha-adrenergic blocker phenoxybenzamine hydrochloride for a period of 5–14 days to control blood pressure preoperatively and to block catecholamine surges during intraoperative manipulation (initial oral dose of 20–30 mg, dose is slowly increased by 10–20 mg per day).
- After satisfactory alpha-adrenergic blockade is established this regimen is complemented by beta-adrenergic blockers such as propranolol at 20–40 mg three or four times daily when cardiac arrhythmia and/or tachycardia persist.

Pharmacological management patients with Cushing's disease

For unilateral adrenalectomy or bilateral subtotal adrenalectomy, administer a single intraoperative dose of 100 mg hydrocortisone, postoperatively, 20–30 mg/day hydrocortisone (+ 0.05–0.2 mg fluocortisone/day) with continuous dose reduction.

Pharmacological management patients with Conn's disease

The aldosterone antagonist spironolactone should be administered at a dose of 200–300 mg/day for 2–3 weeks preoperatively. Potassium may be substituted on the basis of serum electrolyte findings.

INSTRUMENTATION

- Dissection forceps, alternatively bipolar forceps
- Monopolar endo-scissors
- Monopolar and/or bipolar coagulation
- 5 mm multi-clip applicator
- Fan retractor is needed
- Endo-catch bag
- Laparoscopic tower with monitor
- High-flow insufflator (intra-abdominal pressure set at 12–14 cm Hg)
- 0° and 30° 3-chip camera

- Four 12 (10,11) mm trocars, alternatively two 5 mm and two 12 (10,11) mm trocars with optical trocar system provide access to the abdomen.

STEP-BY-STEP OPERATIVE TECHNIQUE

Patient positioning

The patient is placed in the semilateral decubitus position with the side of the lesion elevated at 60° (Figures 12.1 and 12.2). The ipsilateral arm is secured using an arm board and the contralateral arm is fixed beside the trunk and well padded to avoid lesions of neural structures. Alternatively, with the aid of towels wrapped around them, both arms are placed beside the trunk.

At the chest and hip of the non-affected side, two rests support the body when the affected side is elevated. Additional fixation is done using cloth tapes across the hips and the legs. Great care should be taken to pad all rests and cloth tapes generously. When the patient is positioned securely, the table is rolled to a classic flank position 90° to verify the stability of the system.

Camera trocar placement

The table is rolled to 0° to achieve a supine position for entry into the abdomen. After a 12 mm supra-umbilical horizontal skin incision the Veress needle is introduced to insufflate the abdomen for closed trocar placement. The abdominal cavity is insufflated to 12–14 mm Hg using CO_2. Subsequently, the 12 mm camera port is inserted: by using the Visiport system, the 0° laparoscope is placed into the abdominal cavity under vision. After removal of the 0° laparoscope, the peritoneal space is explored with a 30° laparoscope through the 12 mm trocar. Finally, the patient is rolled to the initial semilateral position for additional trocar placement.

Three additional 12 mm trocars are used for a left adrenalectomy. Two trocars are placed along the medioclavicular line. The upper (second) trocar position is 2 cm below the costal margin. The lower (third) trocar position is 8–12 cm below the second trocar. The fourth trocar is placed below the xiphoid at the level of the umbilical camera port (retractor). Alternatively two 5 mm trocars at position three and four for the working instruments and one 12 mm trocar for retraction at position two may be used, since 10 mm instruments (stapler or XXL Hem-lok clips) are only needed in very rare cases.

LEFT LATERAL TRANSPERITONEAL TECHNIQUE

The splenic attachments to the abdominal side wall and the diaphragma are released (Figures 12.3 and 12.4).

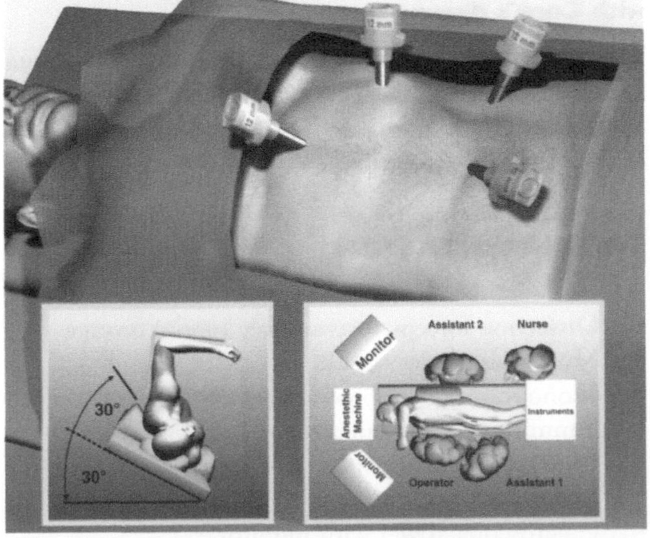

Figure 12.1 Patient positioning, port placement, operating team, and equipment for left-sided transperitoneal laparoscopic adrenalectomy (semilateral position).

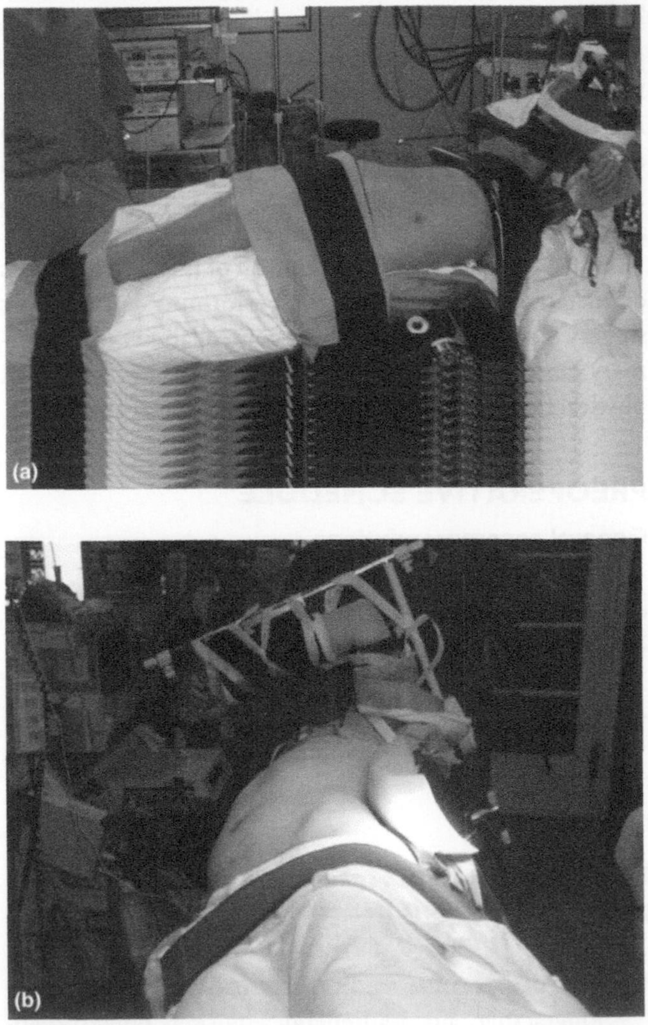

Figure 12.2 Patient positioning for laparoscopic adrenalectomy: (a) right side semilateral position and (b) left side semilateral position.

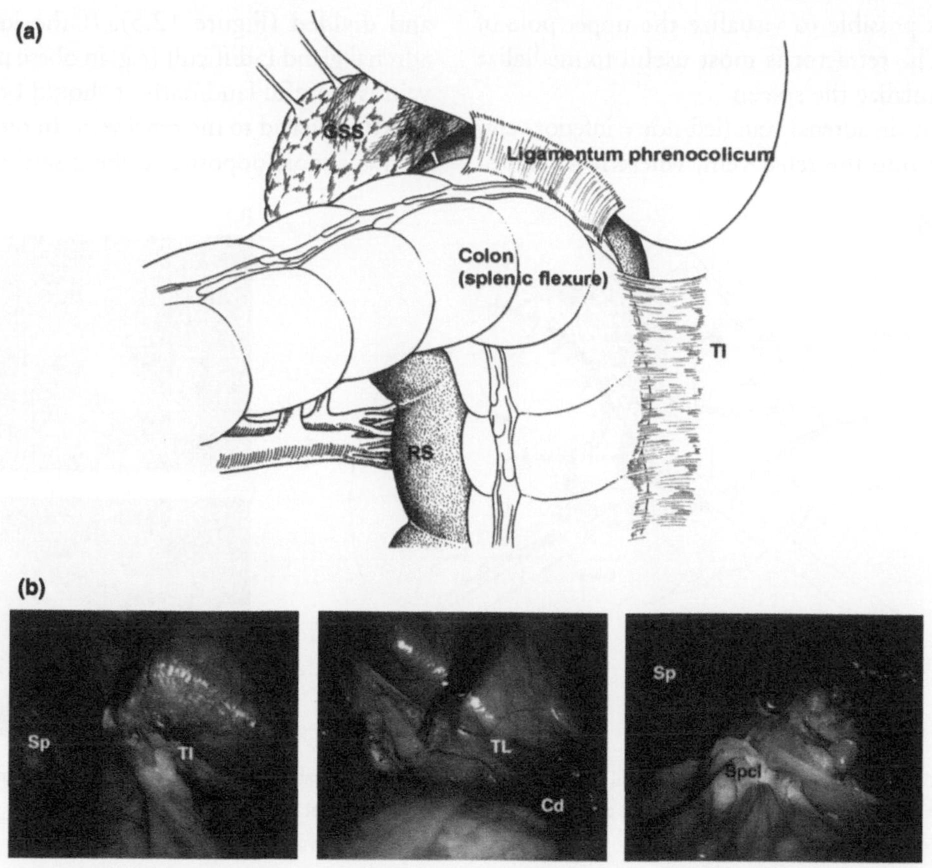

Figure 12.3 (a) Exposure of the splenocolic ligament and of the line of Toldt and subsequent division during left-sided transperitoneal adrenalectomy. (b) Incision of the line of Toldt (cranial left, caudal mid image) with subsequent incision of the phrenocolic. Sp, spleen; Tl, line of Told; Cd, descending colon; Spcl, splenocolic ligament.

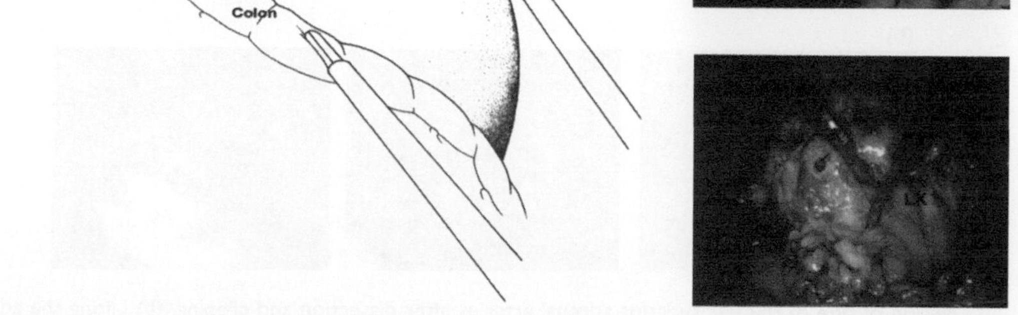

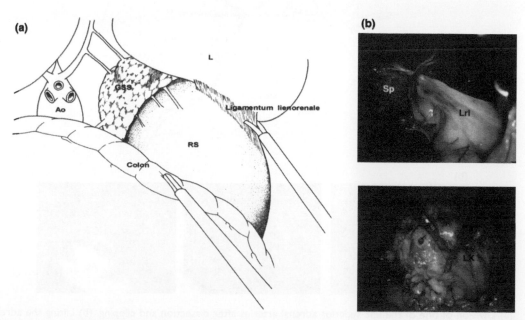

Figure 12.4 (a) Incision of the lienorenal ligament, reflection of the colon medially, exposure and mobilization of the left kidney. (b) Incision of the lienorenal ligament; mobilization of the left kidney. Sp, spleen; LrL, lienorenal ligament; LK, left kidney.

By doing so, it is possible to visualize the upper pole of the left kidney. The retractor is most useful to medialize the colon and cranialize the spleen.

We identify the main adrenal vein (left side = inferior vein) at its termination into the renal vein, where it is clipped and divided (Figure 12.5). If the identification of the adrenal gland is difficult (e.g. in obese patients) the gonadal vein is a useful landmark: it should be identified and followed cephalad to the renal vein. In most cases, the adrenal vein is almost opposite to the insertion of the gonadal in

(a)

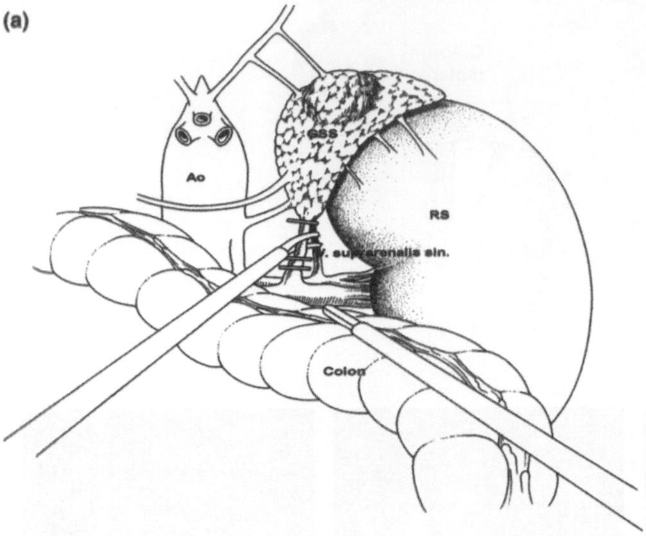

(b)

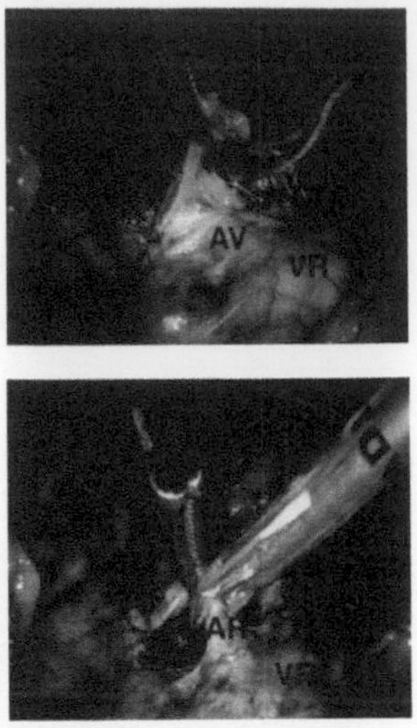

Figure 12.5 (a) Identification of renal and adrenal vein, division of the left adrenal vein after dissection and clipping. (b) Identification of the renal and adrenal vein. The main adrenal vein is clipped and divided. AV, adrenal vein; VR, renal vein.

(a)

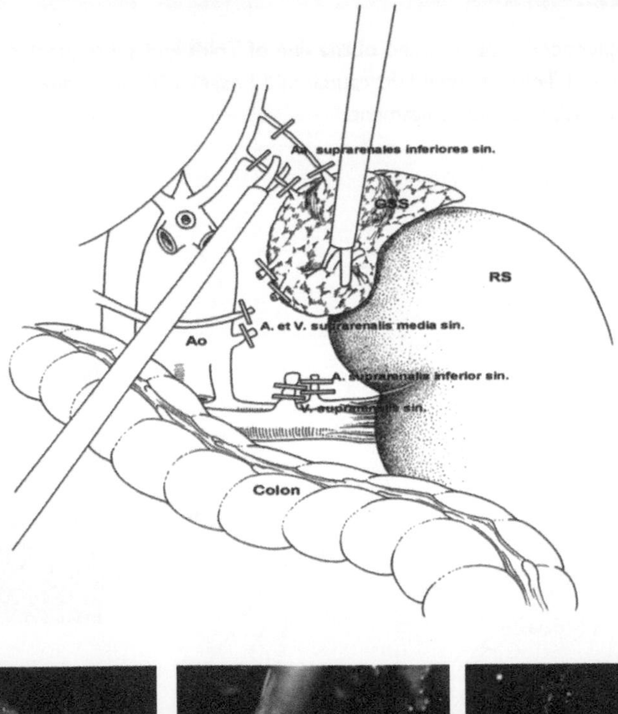

(b)

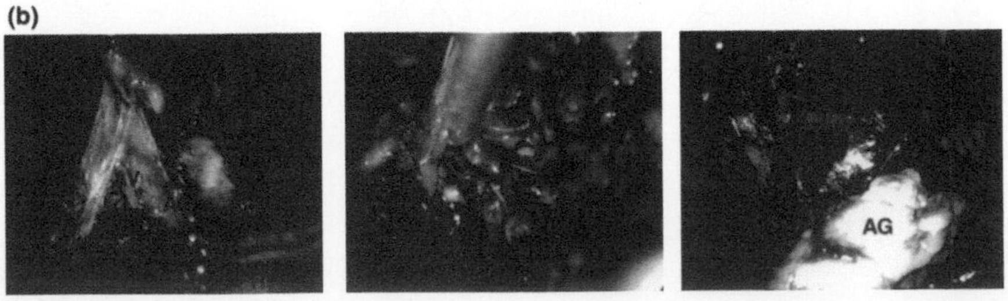

Figure 12.6 (a) Division of one of the left superior adrenal arteries after dissection and clipping. (b) Lifting the adrenal at the venous stump (left). Clipping of one of the left superior adrenal arteries (middle). A second superior adrenal vein is clipped (right). AV, adrenal vein; AG, adrenal gland; RV, renal vein; AA, adrenal artery; AR, renal artery.

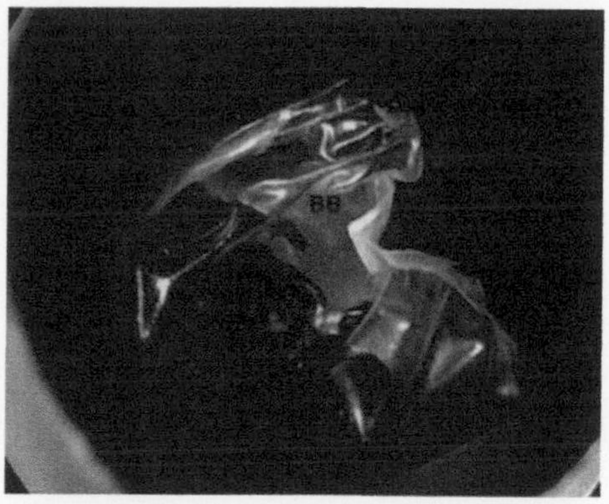

Figure 12.7 Removal of the adrenal gland in the endo-catchbag. BB, ; AG, adrenal gland.

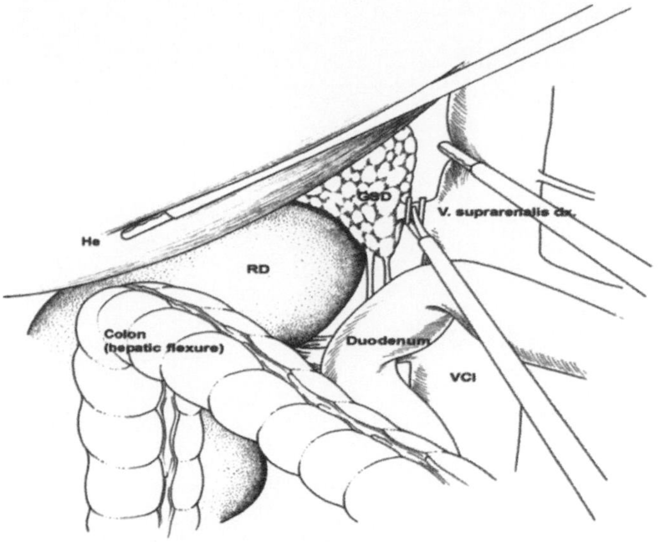

Figure 12.8 Division of the right adrenal vein after dissection and clipping (right laparoscopic adrenalectomy).

the renal vein. The venous stump is used to gently lift the adrenal gland.

We then identify and divide the small medial and superior adrenal vessels (Figure 12.6). The adrenal gland is freed from its lateral and medial attachments.

The specimen is extracted intact in an endo-bag (Figure 12.7). Extraction of the specimen may be performed either via the pararectal caudal trocar site, or alternatively (e.g. for larger specimens) through the camera port, which is extended in an inverse T-shaped incision.

RIGHT LATERAL TRANSPERITONEAL TECHNIQUE

The trocars are placed in a mirror image as for the left-sided adrenalectomy. The liver retractor is inserted by the subxyphoidal trocar. We mobilize and transect the triangular ligament. The liver is carefully retracted cephalad. The posterior peritoneum is transversely incised high along the surface of the liver, extending from the line of Toldt laterally up to the inferior vena cava medial. The duodenum is subsequently mobilized medially to expose the renal hilum. Identification and isolation of the right main (medial) adrenal vein follows. On the right side, the identification and dissection of the hepato-diaphragmal attachments is of utmost importance to be able to lift the liver as far cranially as possible so that the inferior vena cava can be freed almost as far cranially as the insertion of the hepatic veins, to provide optimal exposure of the adrenal gland. In the next step, the adrenal vein is clipped and divided (Figure 12.8). Subsequently, division of the small inferior and superior adrenal vessels separates the adrenal gland from the vena cava. The adrenal gland is entrapped in the sack and removed after complete mobilization.

POSTOPERATIVE SCHEDULE

The skin and fascia closures are performed with absorbable materials after the optimal drain insertion. In some cases no wound drains are necessary.

The most important aspect of postoperative care is the management of the specific endocrinological problems, if any (hormone substitution, but beware of pheochromocytoma!).

Part 3 Laparoscopic Surgery in Childhood

CHAPTER 13

Laparoscopic management of nonpalpable testis

Jan Roigas

INDICATION

In the male population, nonpalpable testis occurs at an incidence of 1% and about 20% of these cases will have a nonpalpable testis.[1] In 1976, Cortesi was the first surgeon to perform laparoscopy for the diagnosis of nonpalpable testis.[2] Today, diagnostic laparoscopy is the gold standard of care for the identification of an intra-abdominal testis.[3] Using the laparoscopic approach it is possible to recognize blind-ending testicular vessels and a blind-ending ductus deferens, a situation that is typical for a vanishing testis and requires no further surgical activity. Also, it is possible to identify testicular vessels and a ductus deferens that are entering the internal inguinal ring. In these cases, an inguinal exploration should be the next surgical step.

When an intra-abdominal testis is identified, either an orchiectomy or a laparoscopic assisted orchiopexy are indicated, depending on the size, appearance, and localization of the testis.

Our technique for a laparoscopic orchiopexy, described here, has been adapted from Mathews and Docimo.[4] Alternatively, if not enough length of the testicular vessels can be achieved by tissue preparation, a laparoscopic one- or two-stage Fowler-Stevens procedure can be considered. The decision to perform a laparoscopic orchiopexy or a one- or two-stage Fowler-Stevens operation is challenging and there are only some aspects that can be helpful, such as the estimation of the distance between testis and internal inguinal ring, the cord anatomy, and the capability of the testis to reach the opposite inguinal ring after mobilization.[5]

An excellent success rate with similar complication rates was reported for laparoscopic orchiopexy.[6,7]

PREOPERATIVE SCHEDULE

- Diet: Patients can have a normal breakfast in the morning, soup for lunch, and fluid only in the evening.
- Bowel preparation: No specific bowel preparation is necessary. Two rectal enemas are administered in the evening.
- Perioperative antibiotic treatment is not necessary.

INSTRUMENTATION

- 1 trocar (5/7 mm)
- 1 trocar (5 mm)
- 1 trocar (5/10 mm)
- 1 trocar (5/10 mm) for scrotal placement
- Optical system (5/7 mm, 0°) for first assistant
- Scissors for surgeon
- Grasper or bipolar grasper for surgeon.

POSITIONING OF THE PATIENT/ OPERATIVE TECHNIQUE

The patient is placed on his back in a 10–20° Trendelenburg position. A catheter has to be placed in the bladder to avoid bladder injury during trocar placement (Figures 13.1–13.3).

Following infra-umbilical incision, placement of the Veress- needle, and establishment of the pneumoperitoneum, three trocars have to be placed.

Beside the first 5 or 7 mm 0° optical trocar at the infra-umbilical site, one 5 mm trocar has to be placed under visual control in the pararectal region on the left side in the middle and slightly above the line between the umbilicus and spina iliaca anterior superior. Similarly, on the right side, a 5 or 10 mm trocar should be placed slightly below this line (Figure 13.4).

After all trocars have been placed the peritoneal cavity should be inspected. Then the patient should be lifted up on the left side and the view should be focused on the operating field.

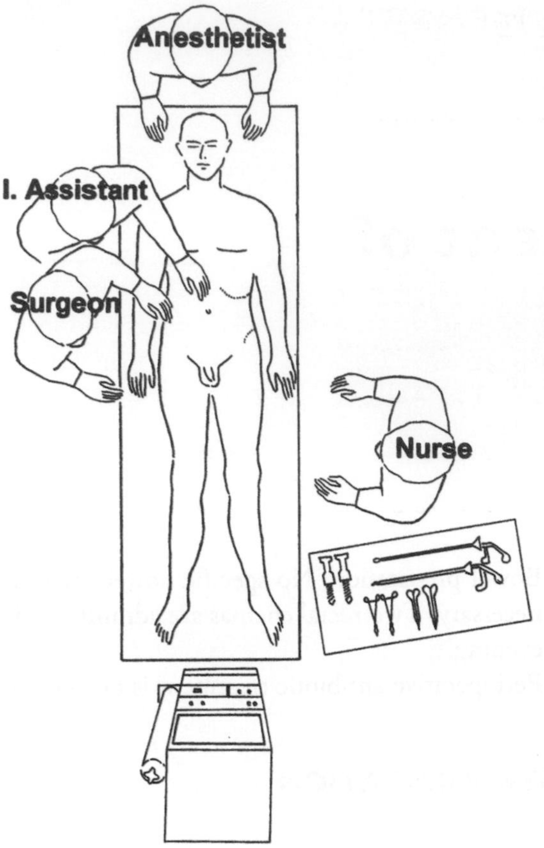

Figure 13.1 Positions of the patient and personnel in the operating room.

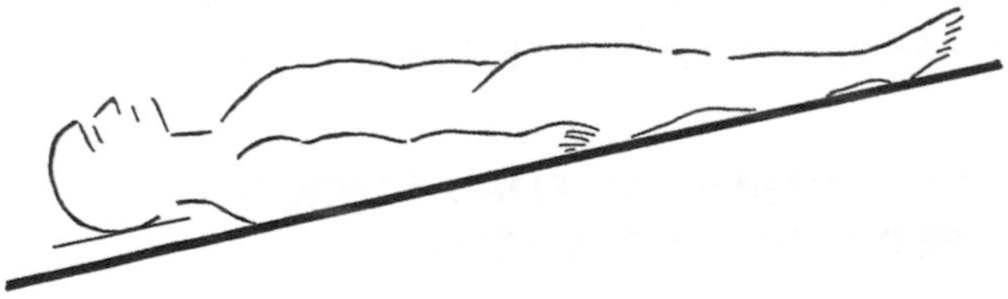

Figure 13.2 The patient is placed in a 10–20° Trendelenburg position.

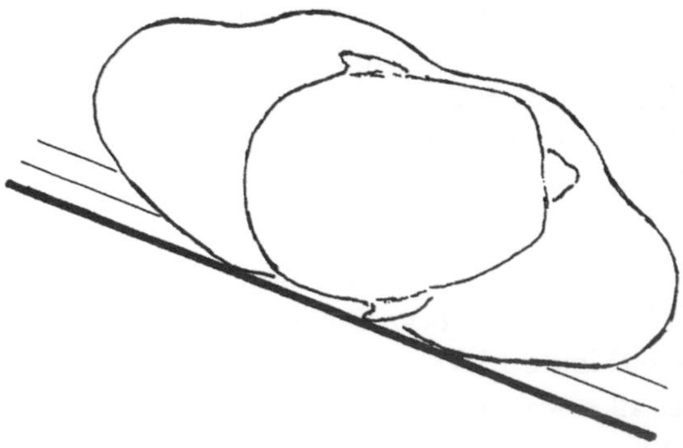

Figure 13.3 After first trocar placement the patient should be lifted up on the left side.

Figure 13.5 demonstrates the important anatomic landmarks; an abdominal testis with the testicular vessels, the ductus deferens, the internal inguinal ring, and the plica umbilicalis lateralis. In this case, a typical situation was

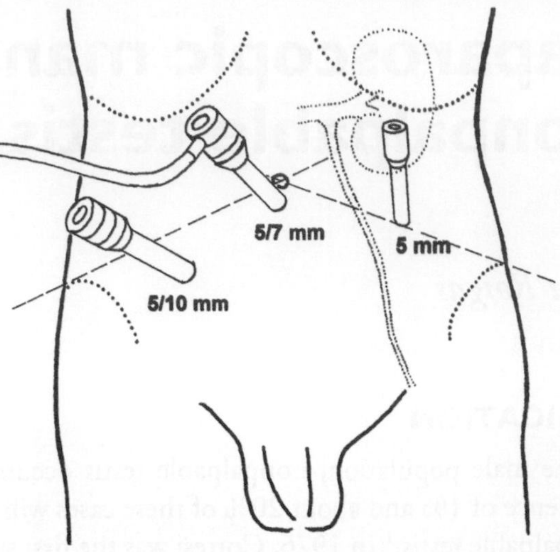

Figure 13.4 The placemenent of the three trocars is as follows: one 5 or 7 mm 0° optical trocar infra-umbilical, one 5 mm trocar on the left side pararectal slightly above the line between the umbilicus and the spina iliaca anterior superior, another 5 mm trocar on the right side slightly below the line between the umbilicus and spina iliaca anterior superior.

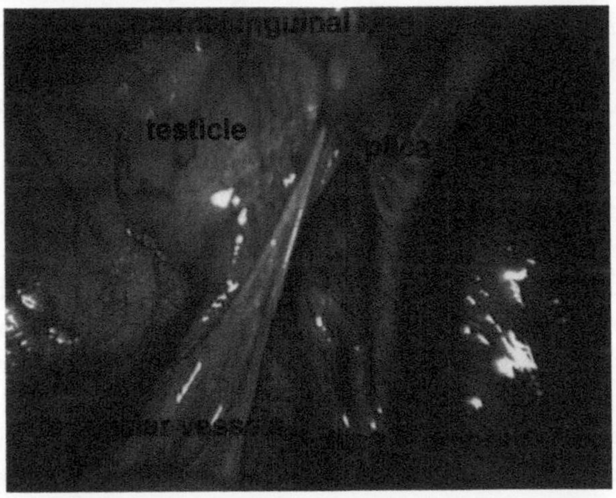

Figure 13.5 After lifting the left side of the patient up important anatomic structures are: colon sigmoideum, internal inguinal ring, testicular vessels, plica umbilicalis lateralis, ductus deferens, and external iliac artery. If an abdominal location of the testis exists, it can be identified along the route of the testicular vessels. In most cases the testicle will be situated close to the internal inguinal ring. In cases where a laparoscopic orchiopexy cannot be performed, the testicle should be separated from the testicular vessels and the ductus deferens. After mobilization, the testicular vessels should be clipped with clips via the 5 or 10 mm lateral port on the right side and transected. The ductus deferens can usually be transected using an electrocautery device, such as a bipolar forceps. The specimen should then be removed via the 10 mm port.

found for the performance of a laparoscopic orchiopexy with the following steps (Figure 13.6):

- careful peritoneal incision around the testis with sparing of the testicluar vessels and ductus deferens with complete mobilization of the testis (Figures 13.7 and 13.8)
- peritoneal incision and mobilization of the testicular vessels and the ductus deferens to achieve mobility of the testis and length (Figure 13.9)
- scrotal incision and trocar placement, enlargement of the incision (Figure 13.10)
- luxation of the mobilized testis into the scrotum (Figures 13.11 and 13.12)
- performance of scrotal orchiopexy using the Shoemaker technique (Figure 13.13).

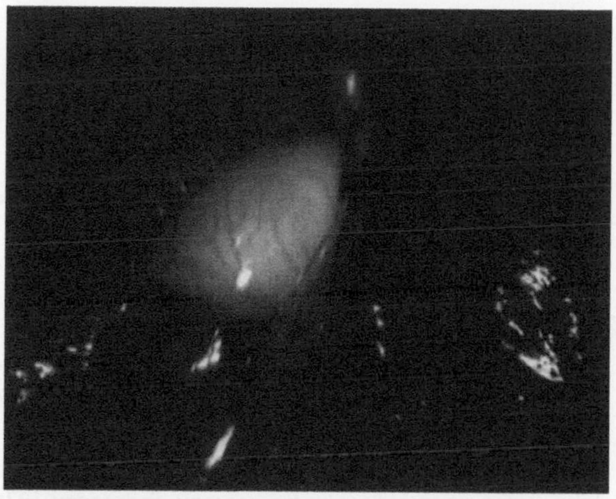

Figure 13.6 If a laparoscopic orchiopexy seems to be possible, the distance between the testicle and the internal inguinal ring should be carefully estimated. Therefore, the testicle should be luxated away from the internal inguinal ring. This allows estimation of the mobility and distance of the testis.

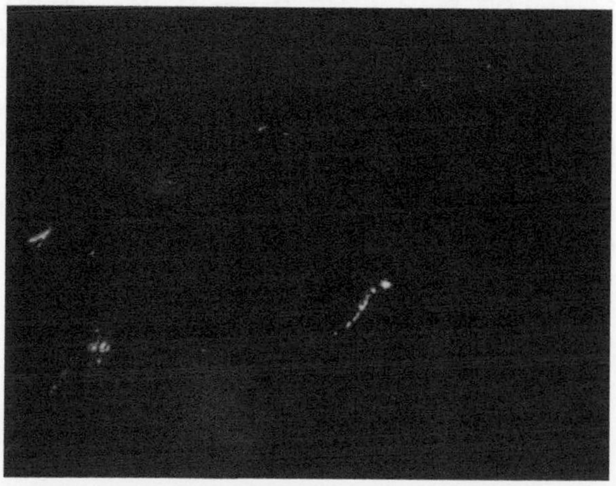

Figure 13.7 The peritoneum should be incised distally from the testicle. This incision should be done very carefully to avoid any damage to the ductus deferens or the testicular vessels.

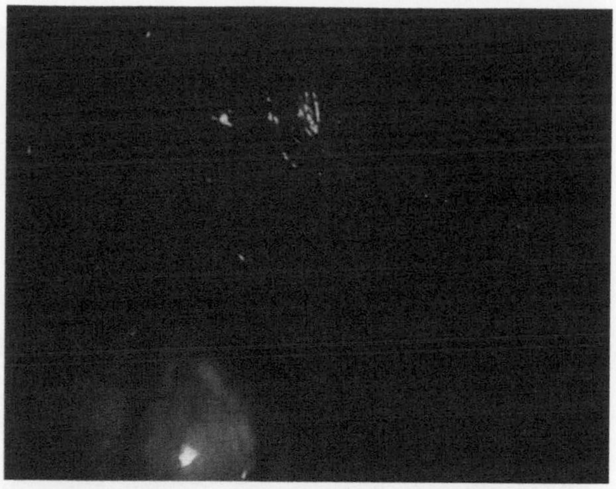

Figure 13.8 Further preparation goes along the ductus deferens in the direction of the seminal vesicle. The ductus deferens with its artery should be completely separated from the surrounding tissue.

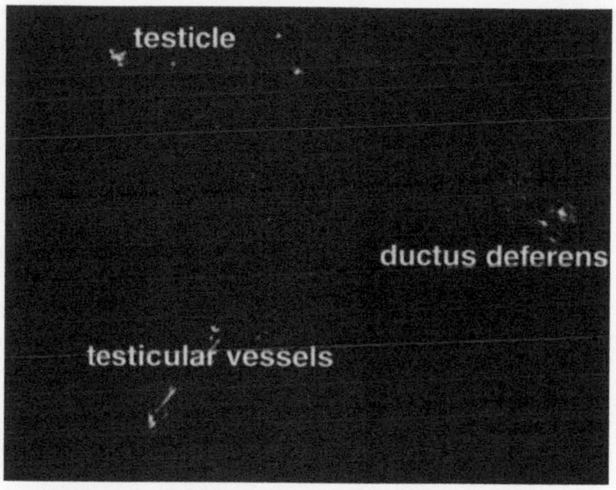

Figure 13.9 The complete separation of the testicular vessels in the cranial direction is the next important step to achieve length. Again, this preparation needs to be done very carefully. Then, the testicle can be lifted up and is completely mobilized. It is only adherent at the ductus deferens and the testicular vessels. Now the surgeon can test whether the testicle can be positioned in the direction of the scrotum.

During the procedure the testicular bundle should be tested for tension and the testis should be inspected. At the end of the operation the adjacent organs should be obeserved for bleeding and the bowel should be inspected for bowel lesions. Usually, it is not necessary to place drainage at the end of the operation.

POSTOPERATIVE SCHEDULE

- Fluid intake 2 hours after surgery
- Yoghurt 4 hours after surgery
- Mobilization on the evening of the operation day

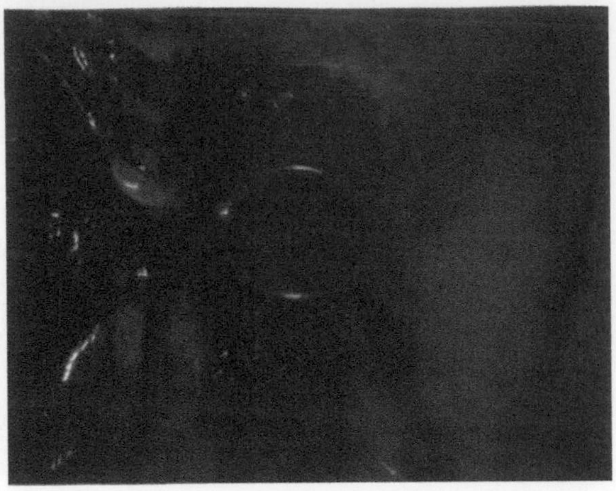

Figure 13.10 A 5 or 10 mm port is placed medially or laterally to the plica umbilicalis into the abdominal cavity via the scrotum. Sometimes in older children or young adults it is helpful to establish a channel using a finger.

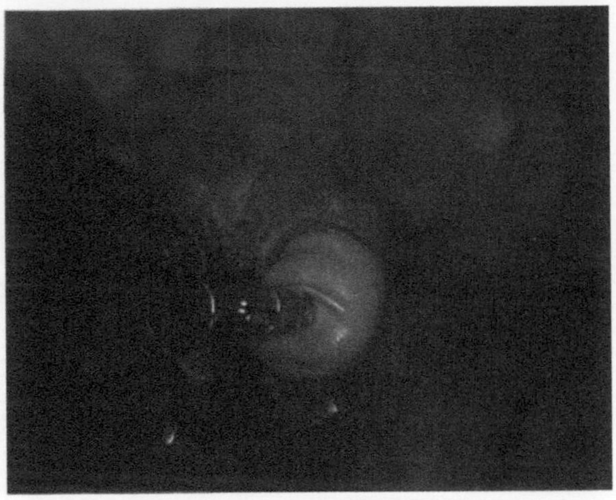

Figure 13.11 A laparoscopic grasper can be positioned via this trocar to the outside and an overhold clamp can then be inserted via the preformed channel into the peritoneal cavity.

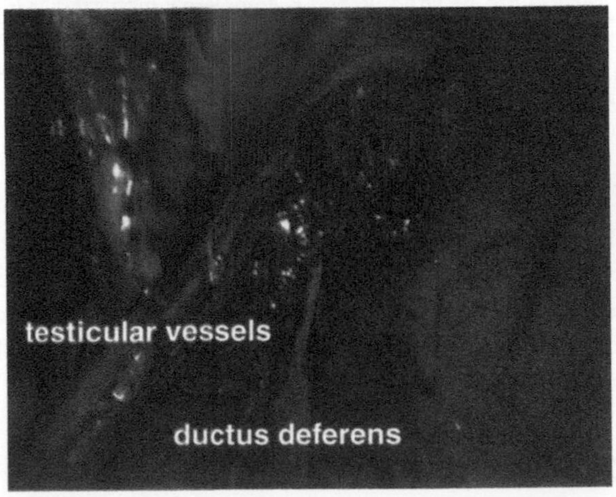

Figure 13.12 With the help of laparoscopic graspers, the testicle is taken by the overhold clamp and brought outside the peritoneal cavity under laparoscopic control and inspected for tension and bleeding.

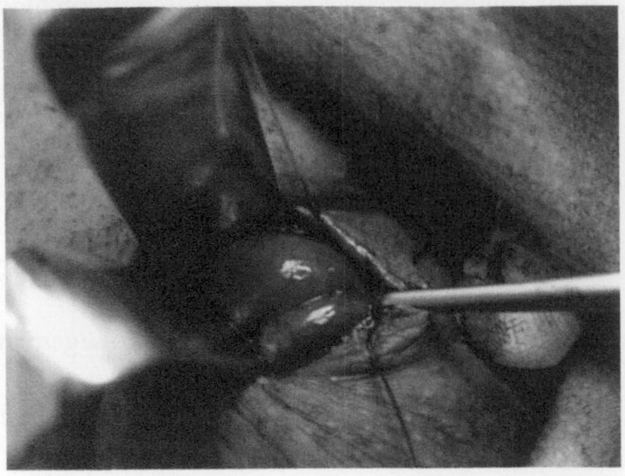

Figure 13.13 The operation is finished following the steps of the standard Shoemaker procedure.

- Regular cost on the first postoperative day
- Pain medication:
  1.5 g methamizole or 1 g paracetamol every 6 hours after surgery
  800 mg ibuprofen twice or 40 drops methamizole/paracetamol at patient's request.

REFERENCES

1. Cryptorchidism: a prospective study of 7500 consecutive male births, 1984–8. John Radcliffe Hospital Cryptorchidism Study Group. Arch Dis Child 1992; 67: 892–9.
2. Cortesi N, Ferrari P, Zambarda E et al. Diagnosis of bilateral abdominal cryptorchidism by laparoscopy. Endoscopy 1976; 8: 33–4.
3. Tekgül S, Riedmiller H, Beurton D et al. Guidelines on pediatric urology. In: European Association of Urology Guidelines, 2007: 8–11.
4. Mathews R, Docimo SG. Laparoscopy for the management of the undescended testis. Atlas Urol Clin 2000; 8: 91–102.
5. Sweeney DD, Smaldone MC, Docimo SG. Minimally invasive surgery for urologic disease in children. Nat Clin Pract Urol 2007; 4: 26–38.
6. Lindgren BW, Darby EC, Faiella L et al. Laparoscopic orchiopexy: procedure of choice for the nonpalpable testis? J Urol 1998; 159: 2132–5.
7. Baker LA, Docimo SG, Surer I et al. A multi-institutional analysis of laparoscopic orchidopexy. BJU Int 2001; 87: 484–9.

CHAPTER 14

Laparoscopic varicocele

Jan Roigas

INDICATION

Laparoscopic varix ligation is a standard laparoscopic procedure. This operation is especially suitable for the less experienced laparoscopic surgeon.

The indications for the minimally invasive or operative treatment of a varicocele can be divided into absolute and relative reasons. According to the European Association of Urology (EAU) guidelines, a reduced testicular size, a pathological spermiogram, a bilateral varicocele, and other factors that influence fertility are absolute indications for operative treatment. Grade two varicocele, recurrent pain, and anxious patients represent relative indications for surgery.

There are several treatment options for the varicocele. Beside the minimally invasive options such as retrograde and antegrade sclerotherapy, the laparoscopic procedure has significantly gained clinical importance during the last years. The classic open surgical techniques (Palomo, Ivanissevich) have been increasingly displaced by minimally invasive treatment options.

The laparoscopic approach to varicocele treatment is very effective, with low rates of recurrence and complications. The most common complication is the formation of hydroceles.[1] Clinical efforts have been made for the intraoperative identification and preservation of lymph vessels that, if completely transected, are responsible for the development of hydroceles. A recent study has shown that the scrotal application of isosulphan blue is helpful during intraoperative preparation of the testicular vein.[2]

From a teaching point of view, laparoscopic varix ligation is ideal for the novice laparoscopic surgeon.

PREOPERATIVE SCHEDULE

- Diet: Patients can have a normal breakfast in the morning, soup for lunch, and fluid only in the evening.
- Bowel preparation: No specific bowel preparation is necessary. Two rectal enemas are administered in the evening.
- Perioperative antibiotic treatment is not necessary.

INSTRUMENTATION

- One trocar (10 mm)
- One trocar (7 mm)
- One trocar (5 mm)
- Optical system (7 mm, 30°) for first assistant
- Scissors for surgeon
- Grasper for surgeon.

POSITIONING OF THE PATIENT/ OPERATIVE TECHNIQUE

The patient is placed on his back in a 10–20° Trendelenburg position. A catheter must be placed in the bladder to avoid bladder injury during trocar placement (see Figures 13.1–13.3).

Following infra-umbilical incision, placement of the Veress needle, and establishment of the pneumoperitoneum, three trocars have to be placed. Patients for varicocele treatment are often young men. Here, the placement of the Veress needle and especially the first trocar can be difficult because of the tension of the musculature of the abdominal wall. It is strongly recommended that good relaxation and a head down position of the patient are secured. In difficult cases, the intra-abdominal pressure can be raised to 18 or 20 mm Hg during the insertion of the first trocar.

Beside the first 7 mm 30° optical trocar at the infra-umbilical site, one 5 mm trocar has to be placed under visual control in the pararectal region on the left side in the middle and slightly above the line between the umbilicus and spina iliaca anterior superior. Similarly, on the right side, a 10 mm trocar should be placed slightly below this line (Figure 14.1).

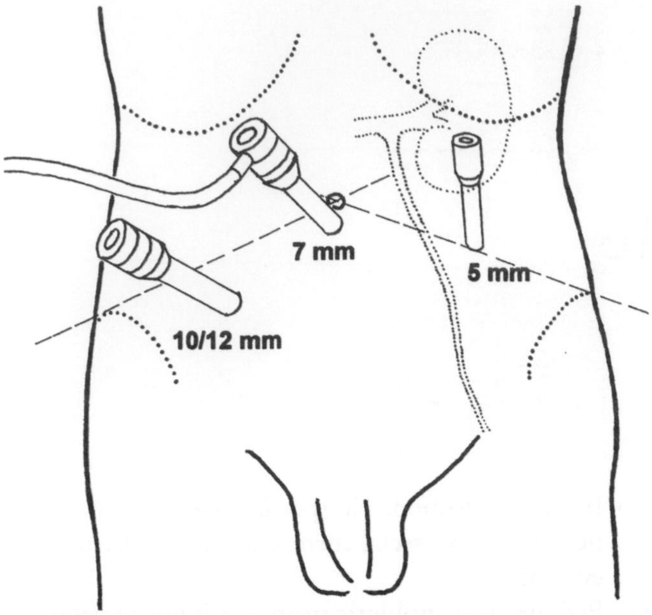

Figure 14.1 The placement of the three trocars is as follows: one 7 mm 30° optical trocar infra-umbilical, one 5 mm trocar on the left side pararectal slightly above the line between the umbilicus and spina iliaca anterior superior, one 10 mm trocar on the right side slightly below the line between the umbilicus and spina iliaca anterior superior.

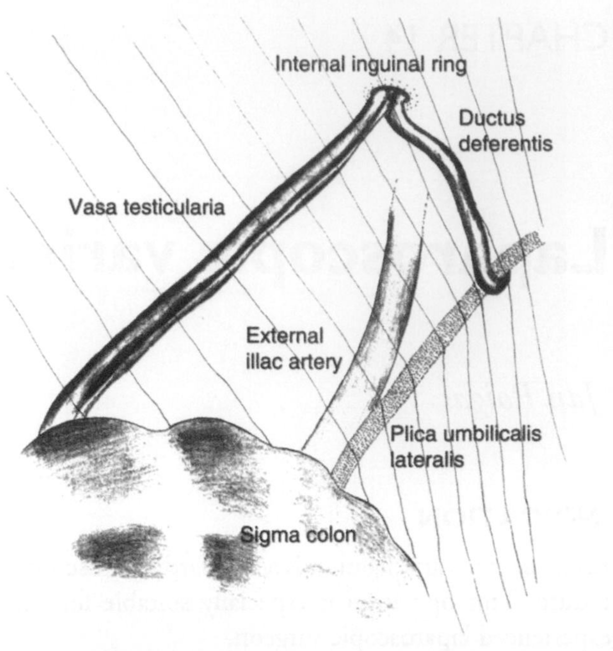

Figure 14.2 After lifting the left side of the patient up important anatomic structures are: colon sigmoideum, internal inguinal ring, testicular vessels, plica umbilicalis lateralis, ductus deferens, and external iliac artery.

When all the trocars have been placed the peritoneal cavity should be inspected. Then the patient should be lifted up on the left side and the view should be focused on the operating field. Figures 14.2 and 14.3 demonstrate important anatomic landmarks, such as the colon sigmoideum, the internal inguinal ring with the testicular vessels, the ductus deferens, and the plica umbilicalis lateralis.

The operation begins, if necessary, with the separation of the mesosigmoid and sigmoid from the lateral abdominal wall without the incision of the parietal peritoneum. Cutting into the mesosigmoid can result in severe bleeding from sigmoideal veins and should be strictly avoided.

Afterwards the peritoneum has to be incised on the medial border of the testicular bundle in the direction of the internal inguinal ring (Figure 14.4). The internal inguinal ring should not be opened, to avoid any injury to the ductus deferens and its artery. With a T-shaped incision (across and lateral to the initial incision) the further preparation of the testicular bundle will be simplified (Figure 14.5).

The bundle is then mobilized from the psoas muscle, without coagulation to avoid injury to surrounding nerves (Figure 14.6). The peritoneum can be separated from the testicular vessels with a laparoscopic sponge until they are completely freed. At this point the surgeon should try to identify and separate the testicular artery and lymph vessels to reduce the postoperative formation of a hydrocele.

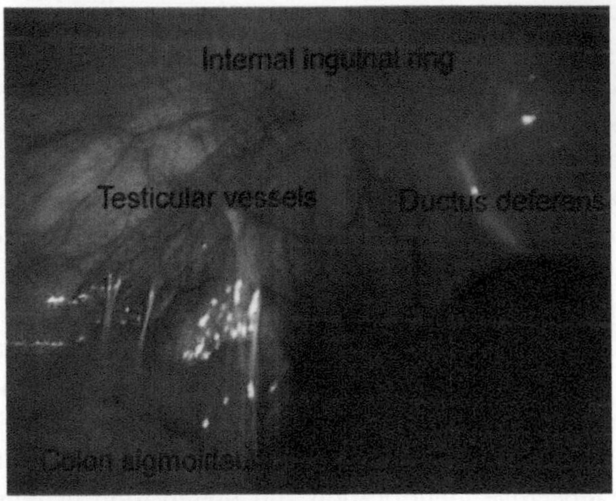

Figure 14.3 Anatomic landmarks should be identified before incision of the peritoneum.

This separation is usually difficult to perform and requires careful inspection and handling of the tissue (Figure 14.7).

Now the testicular veins can be clipped twice using single-use, adsorbable PDS- clips. The clip applicator should be watched carefully to guarantee the closure of the clip (Figure 14.8). After clipping the veins can be transected. Monopolar coagulation should not be applied to stumps of the vessels because of the risk of a thermal injury via the clips (Figure 14.9).

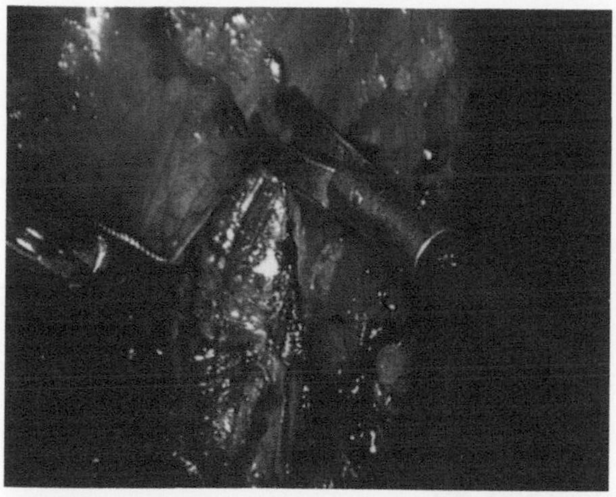

Figure 14.4 Incision of the parietal peritoneum in the direction of the internal inguinal ring. Here, any close contact with the ductus deferens should be avoided. Monopolar coagulation should only be used very carefully.

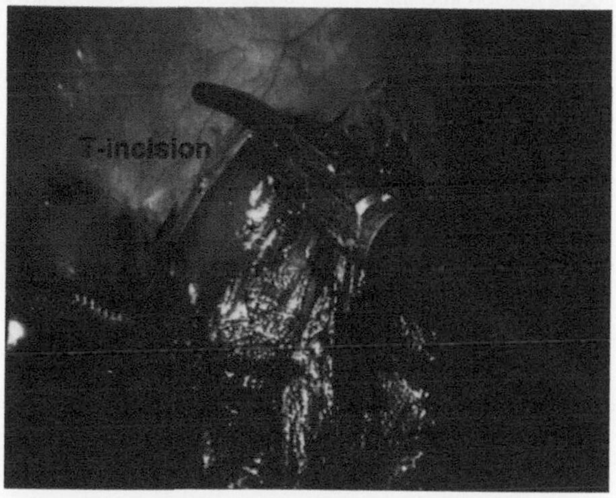

Figure 14.5 A T-shaped incision of the peritoneum allows easier mobilization of the testicular vessels.

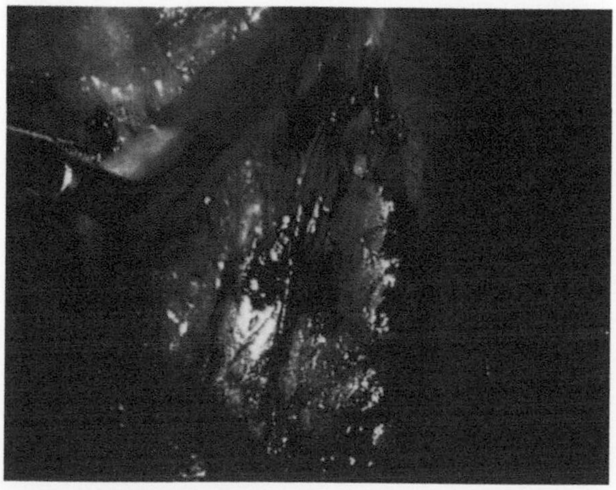

Figure 14.6 With the scissors from the right side, the testicular bundle can be carefully separated.

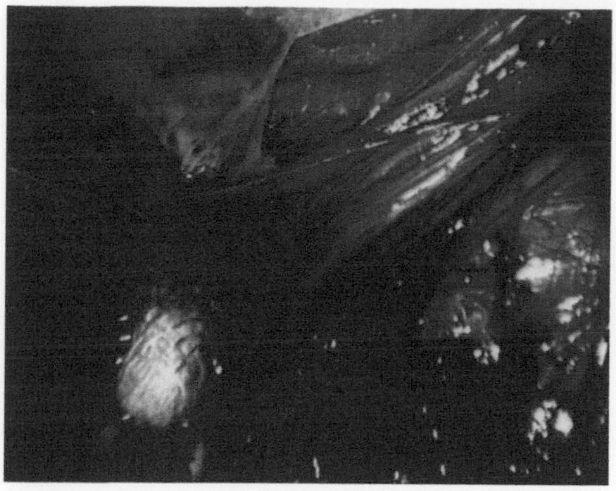

Figure 14.7 The separation of the testicular bundle can be propagated using a laparoscopic sponge.

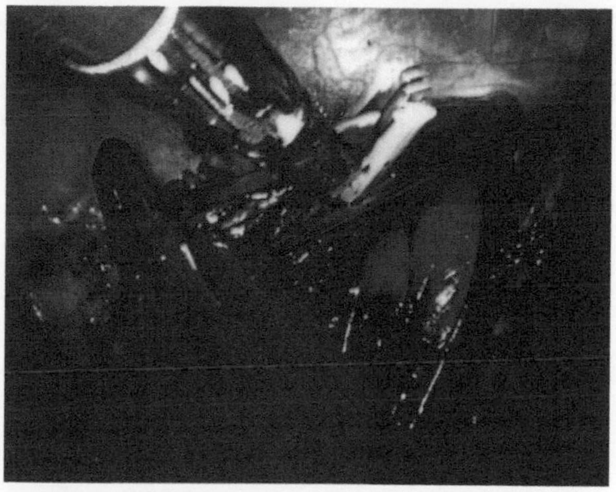

Figure 14.8 If possible, the testicular vein(s) should be separated from the artery and lymph vessels. Then, single-use PDS clips can be placed on the veins.

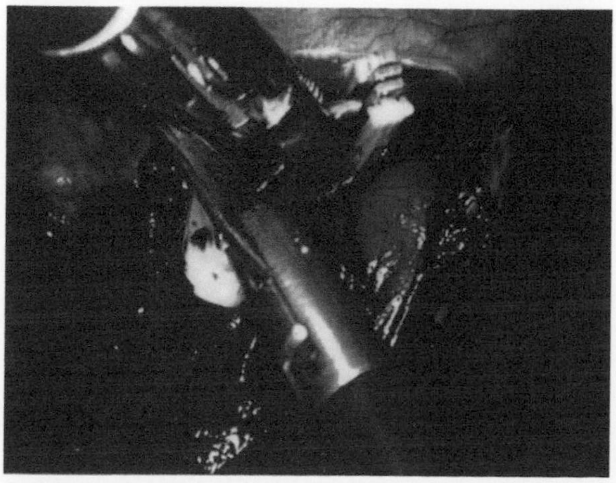

Figure 14.9 Finally the veins are transected with the scissors. No coagulation should be applied.

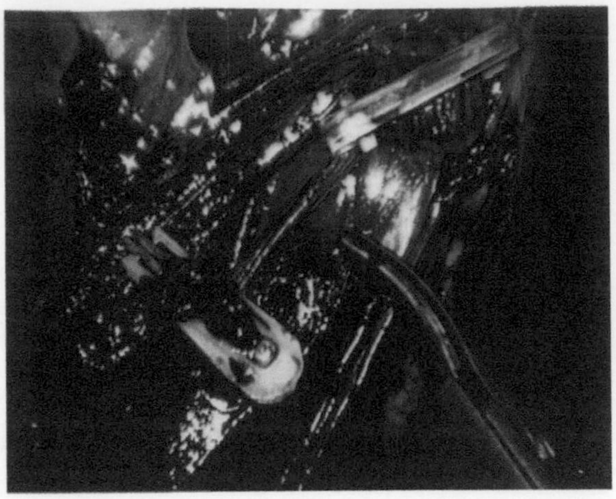

Figure 14.10 After reduction of the intraperitoneal pressure the operating field can be controlled for bleeding.

Finally the operating field should be inspected carefully for bleeding or bowel lesions of adjacent organs (Figure 14.10). Venous bleedings can be better identified if the intra-abdominal pressure is reduced to 5–10 mm Hg. It is not necessary to place drainage at the end of the operation.

POSTOPERATIVE SCHEDULE

- Fluid intake 2 hours after surgery
- Yoghurt 4 hours after surgery
- Mobilization on the evening of the operation day
- Regular cost on the first postoperative day
- Pain medication:
  1.5 g methamizole or 1 g paracetamol every 6 hours after surgery
  800 mg ibuprofen twice or 40 drops methamizole/paracetamol at patient's request.

REFERENCES

1. May M, Johannsen M, Beutner S et al. Laparoscopic surgery versus antegrade scrotal sclerotherapy: retrospective comparison of two different approaches for varicocele treatment. Eur Urol 2006; 49: 384–7.
2. Schwentner C, Radmayr C, Lunacek A et al. Laparoscopic varicocele ligation in children and adolescents using isosulphan blue: a prospective randomized trial. BJU Int 2006; 98: 861–5.

Part 4 Laparoscopy for Female Incontinence

Part 4 Laparoscopy for Female Incontinence

CHAPTER 15

Laparoscopic colpopromontofixation

Alexander Mottrie, P Martens, Renaud Bollens, Peter Dekuyper, Chr Assenmacher, M Fillet, Roland Van Velthoven, and H Nicolas

INTRODUCTION

As the population gets older and aging is a major risk factor for pelvic organ prolapse, the future will be overloaded with a mass of pelvic prolapse repair operations. Many techniques for anterior and posterior vaginal wall repair via vaginal or abdominal approach have been described, all of them with their respective advantages and disadvantages. In this chapter, we describe our minimally invasive technique of laparoscopic colpopromontofixation (LCPF).

The preference for this technique is based on several advantages. With one single access, we are able to correct the three compartments of the small pelvis (anterior, mid, and posterior). Excellent results as to durability and stability can be obtained through the use of prosthetic material. Furthermore, there are the intrinsic advantages of laparoscopy, with excellent overview in the small pelvis, the possibility of a deep dissection, and acceptable postoperative morbidity. Finally, it is a reproducible technique, quick, and relatively easy to perform. The learning curve is quite short (about 20 cases). In case of stress incontinence, this operation can easily be combined with a urethral tape.

As one of the major goals of prolapse surgery is maintenance of or improvement of the patient's urinary, bowel, and sexual function, the patient's desire for preservation of coital, menstrual, and reproductive function should be discussed appropriately before surgery. Informed consent should be given concerning the risk of bowel perforation with the need to stop the procedure, bladder perforation, and vaginal erosion, as well as increase of incontinence or *de novo* incontinence.

INDICATIONS

Any descent of at least one of the three compartments of the vagina – (anterior cystocele, posterior rectocele, and/or dome (uterine descent and/or enterocele) – is an indication for LCPF. It is now generally recommended that all defects of the vaginal wall should be repaired at the same time because occult weakness in other sites could become clinically important. Isolated anterior or posterior defects in older patients may remain an indication for vaginal repair.

In case of stress incontinence, a combined procedure with transvaginal urethral sling is performed.

With modern anesthesiology, there are no real contraindications for this operation. Relative contraindications are history of multiple operations in the small pelvis, severe cardiac failure, and chronic pulmonary obstructive disease (COPD).

PREOPERATIVE PREPARATIONS

Small and large bowel preparation is done the day before surgery with Prepacol®. Urinary infection should always be ruled out. These measures are of extreme importance because a poor bowel preparation or urinary infection can augment the risk for infection of the mesh with consequent problems. Perioperative broad-spectrum antibiotics are administered for 24 hours.

ANESTHESIA

The procedure is performed under general anesthesia. The patient is positioned in a dorsal lithotomy position. An orogastric tube is placed and a bladder catheter indwelled. Anti-embolic stockings are applied. Peroperative Trendelenburg position is needed to get the small bowel out of the small pelvis.

INSTRUMENTATION

Classical laparoscopic materials are needed: two 5 mm ports, one 7 mm port, one 10 mm port, endoscopic grasping forceps, bipolar forceps (Microfrance®), monopolar scissors, and two needle-holders. A multifilament precut polyester mesh (Parietex®) can be used, one approximately 3 cm broad mesh for the anterior, one Y-shaped mesh for the posterior pexy (Figure 15.1). An Ethibond® 2/0 suture with a 3/8 needle is needed for fixation of the prosthesis to elevator muscles and anterior vaginal wall, a Vicryl® 2/0 suture is used for the McCall culdoplasty and closure of the peritoneum. A Pro-Tack® or Ethibond® 0 is used for fixation of both meshes to the promontorium.

OPERATIVE TECHNIQUE

After the patient has been positioned in the Trendelenburg position, the abdomen, perineal area, and vagina are carefully disinfected and draped. A bladder catheter is indwelled.

The surgeon is positioned at the left side of the patient, the first assistant at the contralateral side. A videoscreen is placed at the foot of the bed.

After the pneumoperitoneum has been created (using a Veress needle or open technique), the first 10 mm trocar is introduced just under the umbilicus. A 0° optic lens is used. Now the other trocars are inserted in a diamond configuration. One 5 or 7 mm trocar is inserted on the midline about 3–5 cm above the symphysis pubis. Two 5 mm trocars are inserted on the midclavicular line at the level of the iliac crest (Figure 15.2).

Trendelenburg positioning is carried out up to 25° (Figure 15.3), allowing the bowel to fall out of the small pelvis. If necessary, intra-abdominal adhesions are loosened. The sigmoid is kept away to the left side. This allows opening of the retroperitoneal space at the level of the promontory until the anterior longitudinal ligament is freed, where the mesh has to be fixed at the end of the operation. The medial sacral artery and vein can be spared or coagulated with bipolar coagulation.

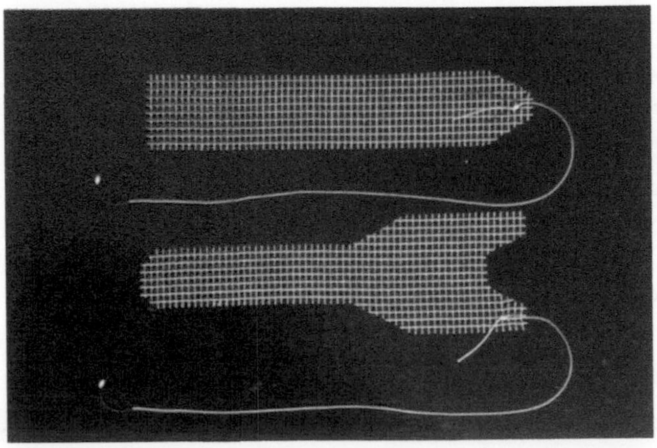

Figure 15.1 Multifilament precut polyester mesh (Parietex®) is used: one approximately 3 cm broad mesh for the anterior and one Y-shaped mesh for the posterior pexy.

Now the right pararectal fold is opened to the level of the ligamentum sacro-uterinum. At the end of the procedure, the mesh is placed and retroperitonealized in this fold.

If the uterus is still in place, it should be fixed to the ventral abdominal wall with a transcutaneous suture (Figure 15.4). In some cases a subtotal hysterectomy is indicated.

As the posterior compartment is done first, the Douglas pouch is opened with a semilunar incision and the posterior vaginal wall and the levator muscles are freed (Figure 15.5). A vaginal wall retractor is sometimes needed to lift the posterior vaginal fornix for easier dissection. To avoid bleeding from hemorrhoidal vessels and possible rectal denervation through excessive dissection of the rectum, we stick to the laterodorsal side of the vaginal wall during dissection.

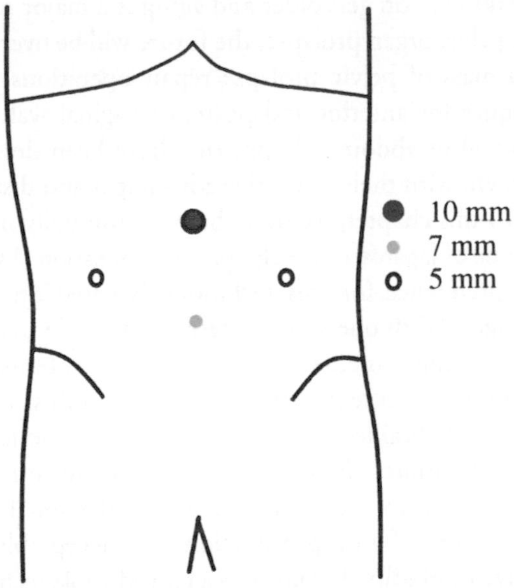

Figure 15.2 Positioning of trocars.

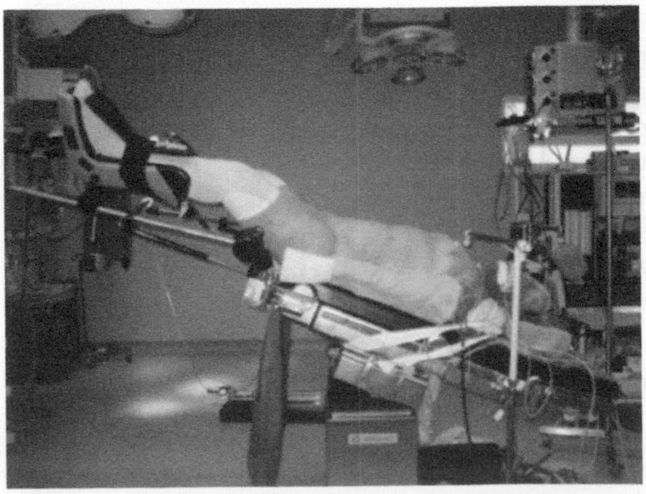

Figure 15.3 A 25° Trendelenburg positioning of the patient is used to allow the bowel to fall out of the small pelvis.

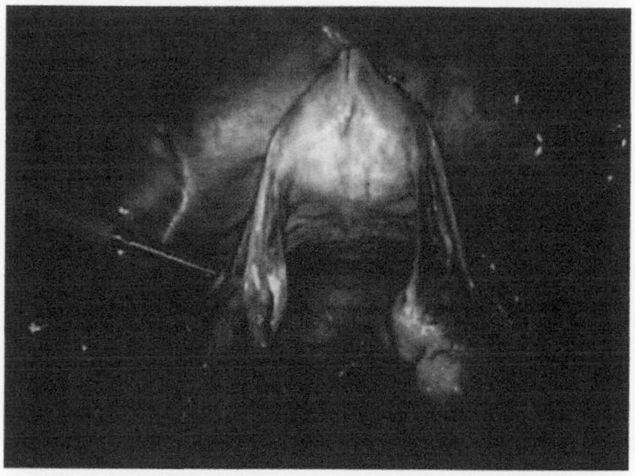

Figure 15.4 Overview with fixation of uterus on abdominal wall to visualize pouch of Douglas.

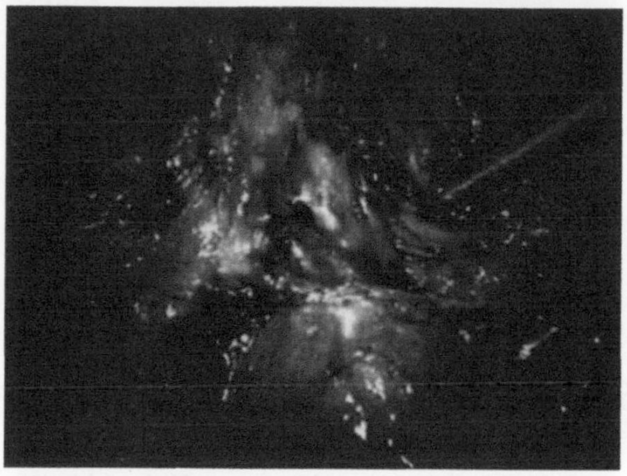

Figure 15.5 Freeing of rectum and pararectal levator muscle.

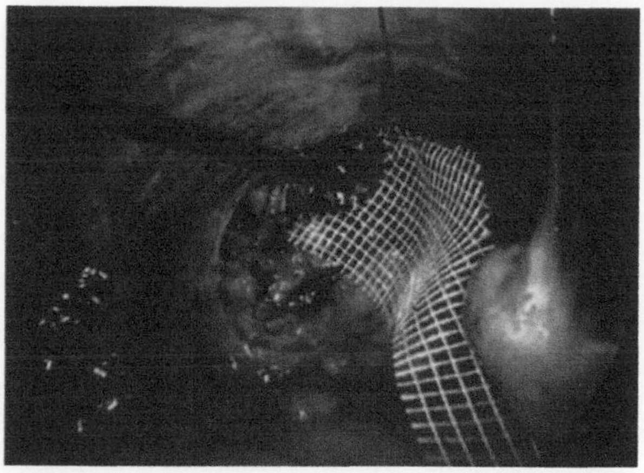

Figure 15.6 Fixation of posterior prosthesis to right levator muscle.

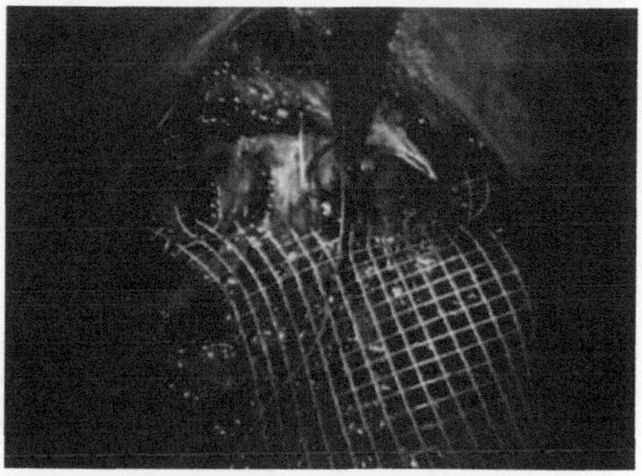

Figure 15.7 The posterior vaginal wall is now fixed with one distal stitch to the prothesis.

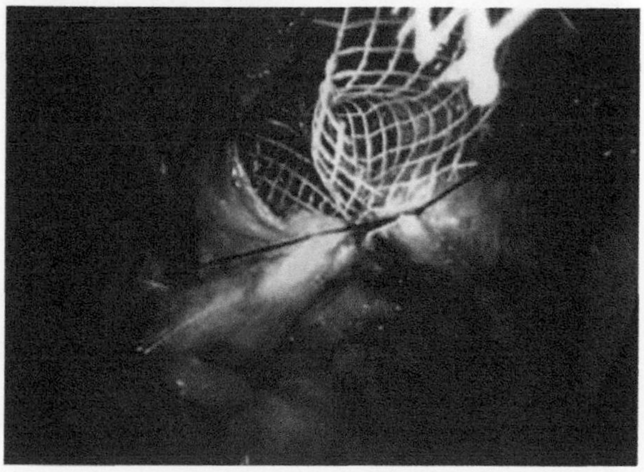

Figure 15.8 Culdoplasty according to McCall.

The posterior prothesis (Y-shaped Parietex) is now introduced in the abdominal cavity via the 10 mm camera port. The two legs of the Y-shaped prothesis are placed over the rectum and tied with an Ethibond suture to the ipsilateral levator muscle (Figure 15.6). The posterior vaginal wall is now fixed with one distal stitch to the prothesis (Figure 15.7).

A culdoplasty according to McCall is then performed. The circumferential suture approximates both uterosacral ligaments, so reinforcing the pouch of Douglas (Figure 15.8). This restores the normal anatomic relationship between the rectum and vagina.

Now, the right-angled retractor is placed on the anterior lip of the vagina to stretch the anterior vaginal wall (Figure 15.9). The bladder is filled with 100–200 ml of saline to improve bladder definition. The peritoneal fold is opened and the vesicovaginal space is entered. The anterior vaginal wall is freed bluntly up to the urethrovesical junction, but not beyond, so as not to disturb innervation of the bladder (Figure 15.10). This is manually controlled with a finger placed inside the vagina. Small bleeders are coagulated with the bipolar forceps. The second mesh is put inside and fixed on the anterior vaginal wall with two running sutures (Ethibond® 2/0) (Figure 15.11). When the uterus is still in place, the running sutures end at the

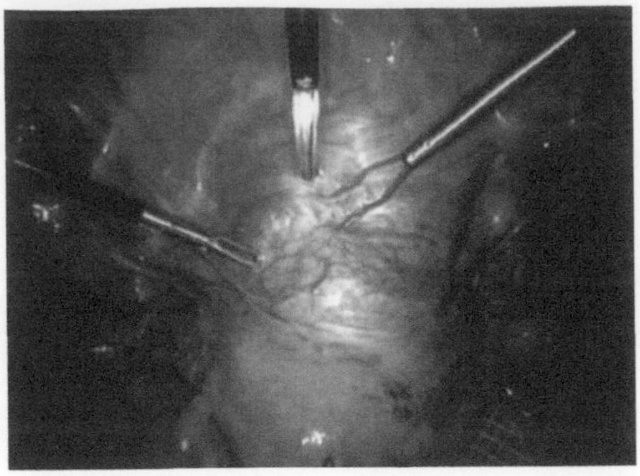

Figure 15.9 Anterior view of cystocele.

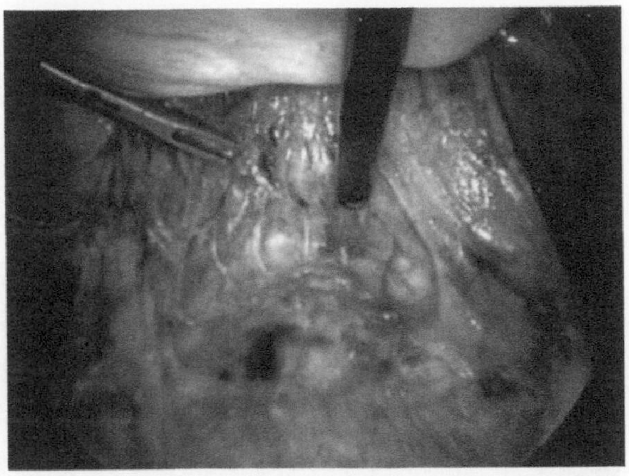

Figure 15.10 Dissection of bladder from anterior vaginal wall to trigone.

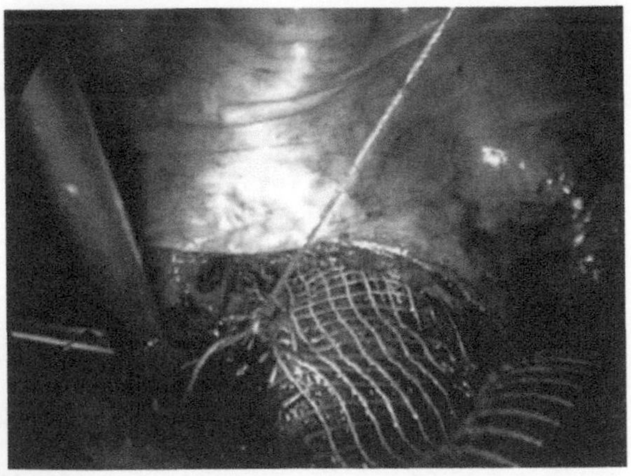

Figure 15.11 Fixation of anterior mesh on vaginal wall with two running sutures.

level of the cervix. The end of the mesh is now put posteriorly through a hole in the right broad uteral ligament (Figure 15.12). Alternatively, it can be cut into two strips that can be pulled posteriorly bilateral of the uterus.

The promontofixation is now performed. The already freed promontory is exposed. The Pro-Tack® is introduced

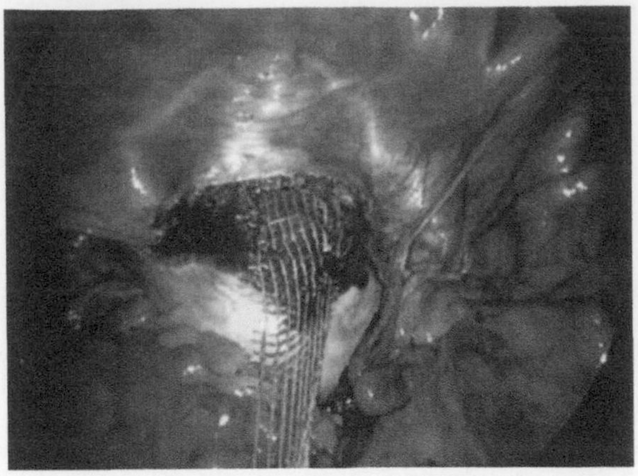

Figure 15.12 View of fixed mesh on anterior vaginal wall.

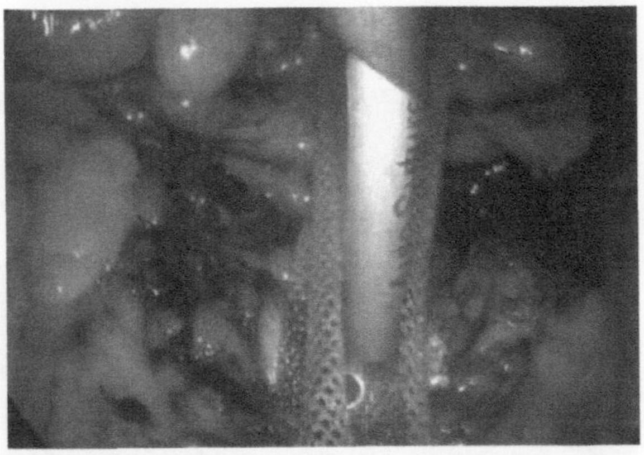

Figure 15.13 Fixation of meshes to promontory with several tacks.

through the medial suprapubic trocar. This tacking device utilizes a helical coil of 3.9 mm in diameter to achieve secure fixation. The forceps grasps the posterior mesh, which is tightened over the promontory and fixed on the promontory with two tacks. Now, the anterior mesh is grasped and pulled over the promontory. Several tacks are inserted through the mesh into the periosteum and the anterior longitudinal ligament (Figure 15.13). Excess mesh is cut away and removed (Figure 15.14). As an alternative to the tacker, both meshes can be fixed using a nonresorbable suture.

Finally, retroperitonealization is performed with Vicryl® 2/0 running suture.

PEROPERATIVE COMPLICATIONS AND POSTOPERATIVE CARE

No wound drain is left in place. Peroral nutrition starts on the first postoperative day. The bladder catheter is removed on the second postoperative day. The patient is discharged once micturition and defecation functions are restored, usually on the third postoperative day. Complications are rare. When bladder perforation occurs, the defect

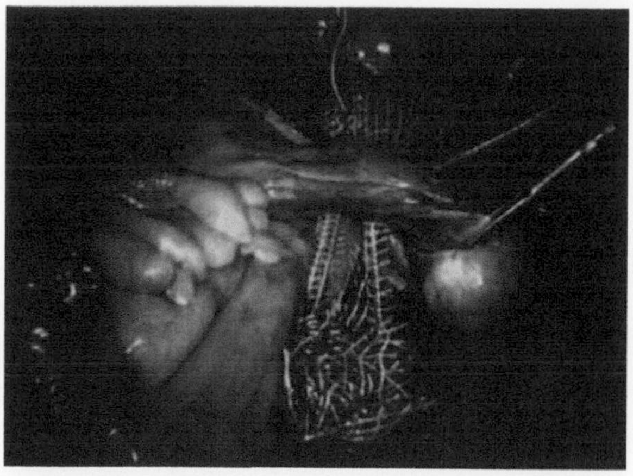

Figure 15.14 Overview of the two meshes fixated on the promontory.

is closed with Vicryl® 2/0 and the catheter is first removed on the fourth postoperative day. Vaginal perforation is closed in two layers to secure a water-tight repair. Broad-spectrum antibiotics are continued for 48 hours. In bowel perforation, the defect is closed with Vicryl® 3/0. The procedure is aborted. No prosthesis is left behind.

RESULTS

There are excellent anatomical results (> 95% of cases have no recurrence). As to functional results, the stress incontinence rate depends on whether the technique is combined with a transvaginal urethral sling. If there is no sling, *de novo* stress incontinence is estimated to be 20%, and is easily resolved by putting in a transvaginal urethral sling. Bladder instability improves or disappears in 60%. As to obstipation, a typical preoperative complaint in these patients, only a minority encounters ameliorization. It is believed that the obstipation is symptomatic of an intraluminal bowel problem rather than an obstructive problem.

CONCLUSION

We believe that this technique fulfils the basic principles of pelvic reconstructive surgery for the following reasons:

- there is repositioning of different organs with respect to their anatomic relationship
- there is repair and/or preservation of urinary and anal continence
- there is preservation of satisfying sexual activity
- it achieves a durable result
- it is minimally invasive.

BIBLIOGRAPHY

Deval B, Fauconnier A, Repiquet D et al. Surgical treatment of genitourinary prolapse by the abdominal approach. Apropos of a series of 232 cases. Ann Chir 1997; 5(3): 256–65.

Reddy K, Malik T. Short-term and long-term follow-up of abdominal sacrocolpopexy for vaginal vault prolapse: initial experience in a district general hospital. J Obstet Gynaecol 2002; 22(5): 532–6.

Von Theobald P. Laparoscopic promontofixation. J Chir 2001; 138(6): 353–7.

Wattiez A, Canis M, Mage G, Pouly JL, Bruhat MA. Promontofixation for the treatment of prolapse. Urol Clin North Am 2001; 28(1): 151–7.

Part 5 Laparoscopic Surgery on Prostate/Urinary Bladder

CHAPTER 16

Robotic surgery in urology – robotic-assisted radical prostatectomy

Andreas H Wille

INTRODUCTION

During recent years the use of robotic-assisted approaches has been growing as an attractive option in minimally invasive surgery. Intuitive Surgical Inc. (Sunnyvale, CA, USA) and Computer Motion (Santa Barbara, CA, USA) were the companies that initially developed the technology for robot-assisted surgery, attempting to overcome the limitations of traditional laparoscopic techniques. The technical developments led to highly sophisticated, reliable tools, and have influenced almost all fields of surgery.

Robotic-assisted laparoscopic techniques have emerged, allowing surgeons to more readily overcome the difficult learning curve[1] and shorten operative times for such minimally invasive abdominal and pelvic operations.[2,3] Certainly, the device eases the technical challenge of intracorporeal suturing and may make reconstructive laparoscopic procedures more accessible to surgeons without extensive laparoscopic experience. Taking this into account, the development and dissemination of robotic surgical tools, such as the da Vinci system, have the potential to alter the way urologists approach complex laparoscopic procedures like pyeloplasty or cystectomy with urinary diversion.[4,5]

Robotic-assisted radical prostatectomy (RARP) involves performing a laparoscopic radical prostatectomy using a robotic interface. This approach is now widely accepted and reliable data are available.[6,7] Today, the most commonly used robotic system in urology is the da Vinci Surgical System™ (Intuitive Surgical). This intuitive master–slave system provides the surgeon with 3D imaging that adds to precision and dexterity while performing the operation. Additional benefits are the wristed instruments with 7° of freedom, tremor-filtering and scaling of movements, intuitive finger-controlled movement, and last but not least, reduced surgeon fatigue due to the improved ergonomics.[8]

Robotic-assisted prostatectomy is viewed as the most natural application, as the small-wristed instruments and the magnified 3D view have significant advantages in pelvic surgery. The new generation of the robotic system (da Vinci™ S) is a four-arm system and combines some improvements such as easier handling, greater mobility of the instrument arms, and better vision (e.g. high definition).

ROBOTIC PROSTATECTOMY STEP-BY-STEP

Technique

The method is described for the da Vinci™ standard three-arm System (Figure 16.1) and is performed transperitoneally based on the laparoscopic technique with several modifications. In contrary to the pure laparoscopic technique the mobilization of the seminal vesicles is done after the bladder neck is dissected.

Surgical steps

- Mobilization of the bladder
- Incision of the endopelvic facia and preparation of the lateral aspect of the prostate and the apex
- Ligation of the dorso-venous complex (DVC)
- Preparation and dissection of the bladder neck
- Mobilization of the seminal vesicles
- Dissection of the pedicles or nerve sparing procedure
- Dissection of the apical urethra
- Vesico-urethral anastomosis

Preoperative Schedule

(see chapter Laparoscopic Radical Prostatectomy)

Anaesthetic Regimen

(see chapter Laparoscopic Radical Prostatectomy)

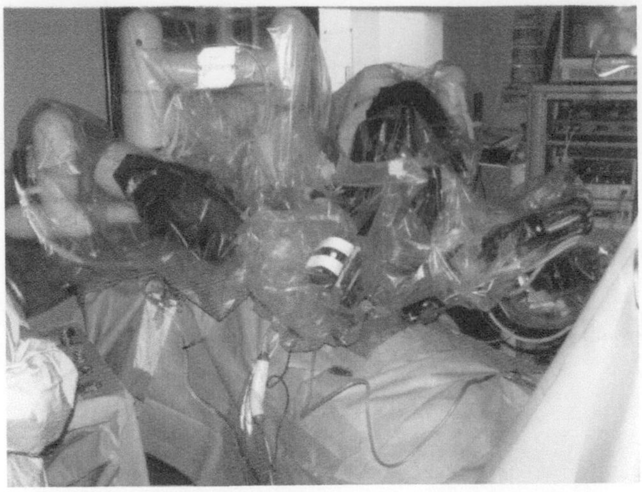

Figure 16.1 Set-up of the robot arms and positioning of the patient.

Instrumentation

8 mm da Vinci™-Instruments
EndoWrist®Permanent Cautery Hook Instrument*
EndoWrist®Curved Scissors*
(*alternatively a EndoWrist®HotShears™ monopolar scissors can be used)
EndoWrist®Bipolar Forceps (optional: Maryland Bipolar Forceps)
Large Needle Driver (2)
additional: *ProGrasp* Forceps for heavy retraction

Laparoscopic Instruments

Suction device «Elefant» (Porges, France)
Reticulating Fanned Endoretractor
Overholt clamp (Aesculap, Gemany)
Atraumatic grasper (Aesculap, Gemany)
Needle Driver (Aesculap, Gemany)
Hem-o-Lock Clip applicator (Weck Closure Systems, USA)

Sutures and Clips

2×0 Vicryl, SH needle
3×0 PDS, RB-1 needle
10 mm Hem-o-Lock Clips (Weck Closure Sytems, USA)

Port placement

The Veress needle is inserted in the left upper quadrant of the abdomen to establish the pneumoperitoneum. After insufflation is completed an incision is made directly above the umbilicus and a 12 mm camera port is inserted. Two 8 mm da Vinci™ ports are set inferior to the umbilicus about 8 cm away from the midline. These ports and the operating field should form an equilateral triangle. It is important to follow these geometric considerations to give the instruments the necessary space and mobility. Two assistant ports are inserted laterally, 2–3 cm above the midpoint between the da Vinci™ ports and iliac spine (W-shape setting). An additional 10 mm port is inserted between the ports on the right side, 2–3 cm above the optical port (Figures 16.2 and 16.3). A 0° lens is used for the entire procedure.

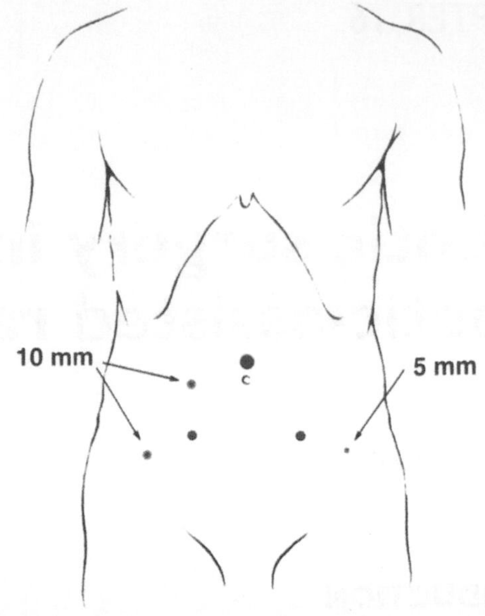

Figure 16.2 Port positions for robotic prostatectomy.

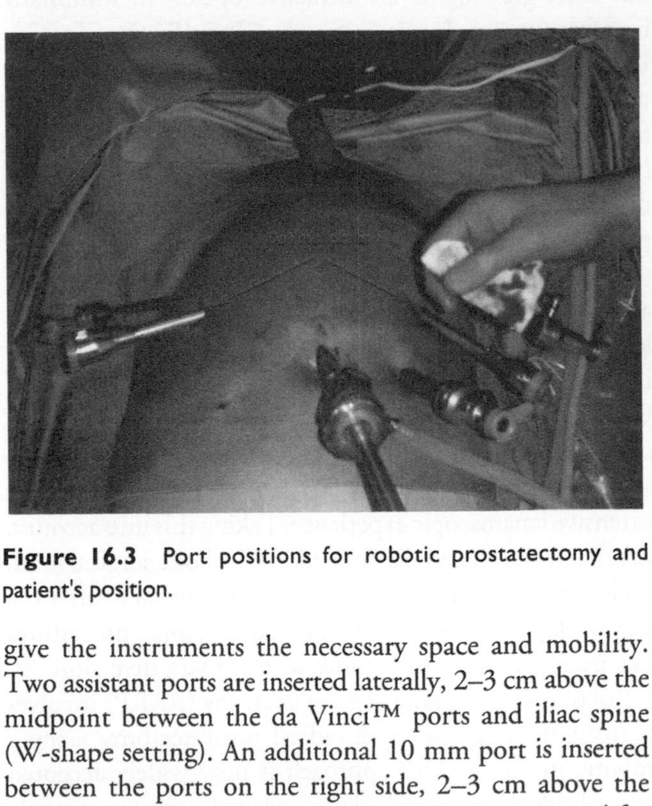

Figure 16.3 Port positions for robotic prostatectomy and patient's position.

Incision of the peritoneum and bladder mobilization

The instruments used are:

- Right arm: electric hook (monopolar scissors)
- Left arm: bipolar forceps
- Assistant: suction, retractor or forceps.

A transverse peritoneal incision is made, cutting the medium umbilical ligament. The excision is continued laterally to the vasa at either side and the pubic bone is exposed. Counter traction of the peritoneum is achieved with the bipolar forceps; bowel retraction is maintained with a fan retractor by the assistant. To improve bladder mobility the vasa are dissected, if necessary. The anterior bladder wall is mobilized until the endopelvic fascia and the prostate are exposed up to the base.

Opening the endopelvic fascia

The instruments used are:

- Right arm: electric hook (monopolar scissors)
- Left arm: bipolar forceps
- Assistant: suction, retractor or forceps.

The endopelvic fascia is opened, exploring the prostate from the bladder neck to the apex. The apical preparation is completed at this step; the dorsal venous complex (DVC) and the urethra are visualized (Figure 16.4).

Ligation of the dorsal venous complex

The instruments used are:

- Right/left arm: needle driver
- Assistant: grasper/suction; scissors.

Different types of sutures are possible, we use a 2×0 Vicryl with an SH needle. The needle is inserted behind the DVC at a right angle and pushed around the apex by turning around. For safety reasons the stitch is repeated and the suture is tied tightly (Figure 16.5).

Anterior bladder neck preparation

The instruments used are:

- right arm: electric hook (monopolar scissors)
- left arm: bipolar forceps
- assistant: suction, grasper.

The covering fat tissue is removed and the bladder neck is identified. Moving the catheter back and forth can help to define the junction between bladder and prostate by watching the catheter balloon. The ventral aspect of the bladder neck is incised similar to the laparoscopic approach (see Chapter 18) (Figures 16.6–16.8).

Different techniques for preparation have been published. We always prefer a careful, bladder neck preservation, making bladder neck reconstruction unnecessary in most cases (Figures 16.6 and 16.7).

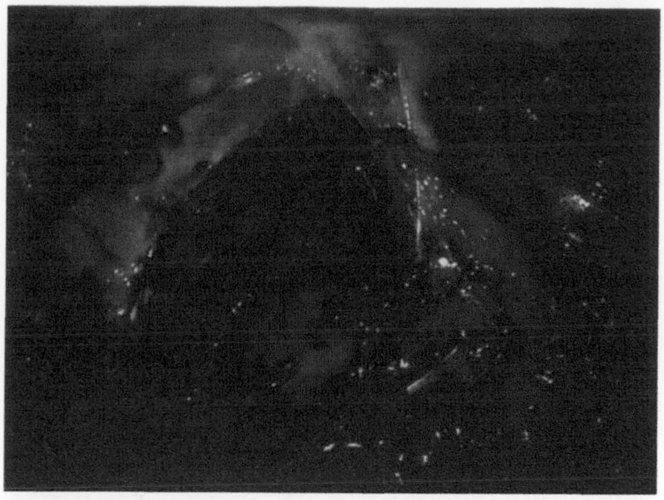

Figure 16.4 Incision of the endopelvic fascia on the left side, showing the left puboprostatic ligament.

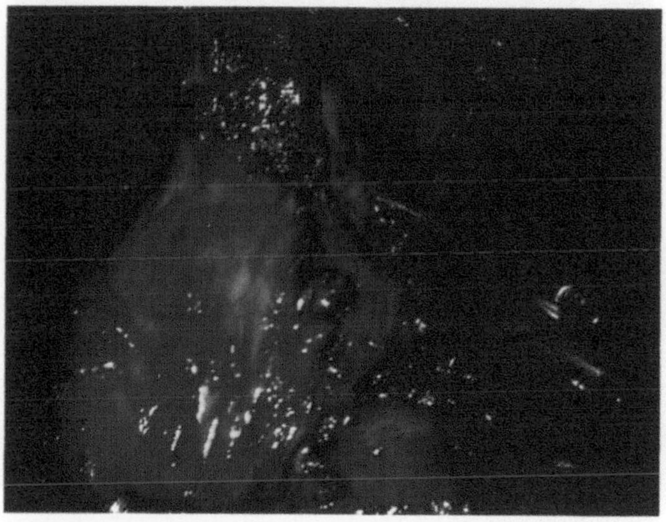

Figure 16.5 A large CT1 needle is used for ligation of the dorsal-venous complex.

Note: switching to a 30° face-down lens may be helpful at this point and for the following steps.

Posterior bladder neck and seminal vesicles

The instruments used are:

- Right arm: electric hook (monopolar scissors)
- Left arm: bipolar forceps
- Assistant: suction, grasper.

Once the ventral urethra is incised the catheter is pulled through the incision and lifted upwards, while the

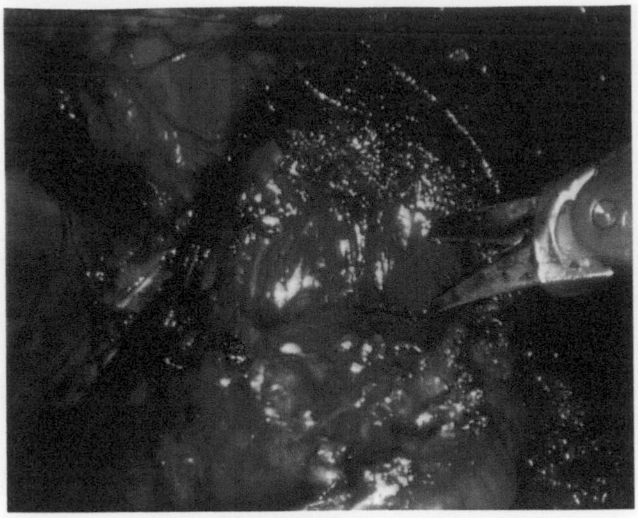

Figure 16.6 The anterior aspect of the bladder neck is incised and the junction between urethra and bladder is exposed.

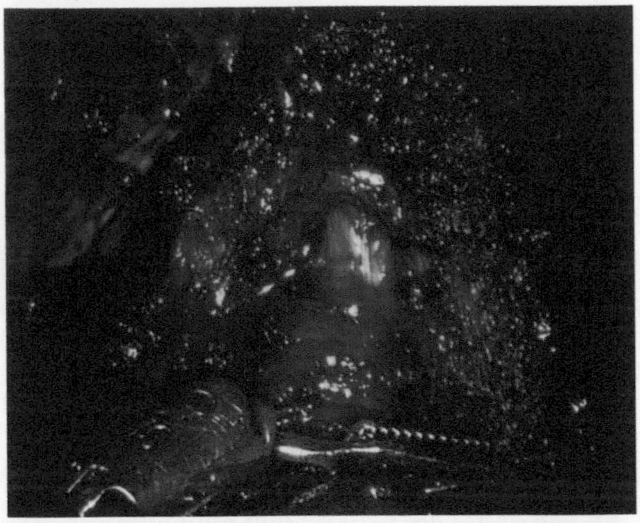

Figure 16.7 Division of the anterior bladder neck continues laterally exposing the circumference of the prostatic urethra.

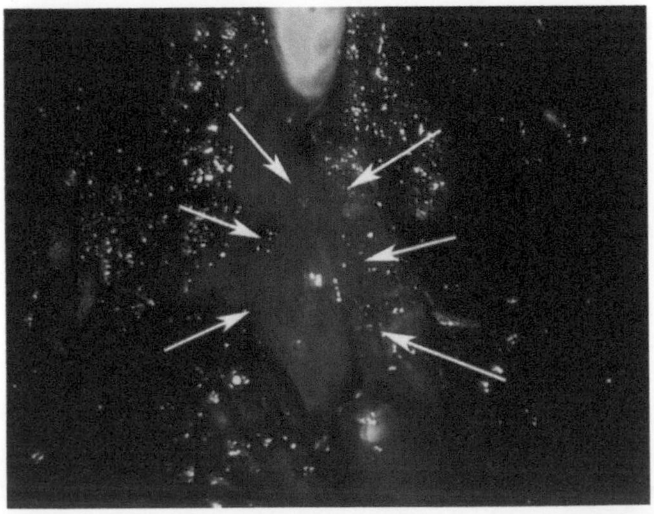

Figure 16.8 The bladder neck is opened; the catheter lifted up to pull the prostate upwards to expose the dorsal aspect of the bladder neck. (arrows show bladder neck).

external part of the catheter is immobilized with a clamp. After the entire prostate is lifted up the dorsal aspect of the bladder neck is incised and pulled gently downwards with the bipolar grasper. Preparation is continued straight downwards, keeping the full thickness of the dorsal bladder neck intact. This part is most challenging because the correct plane between prostate and bladder neck can easily be missed.

Note: the direction of the preparation is crucial for identifying the right layer. Going in at a flat angle will result in entering the prostate and missing the seminal vesicles. Going in too steeply may affect the bladder trigonum.

After the posterior aspect of the bladder neck is completely dissected the vasa and seminal vessels can be identified. The facial layer is incised, the vasa are cut, and their inferior portion is lifted up by the assistant to expose the seminal vesicles. The vesicles are mobilized and supplying vessels are clipped or coagulated using bipolar current. Now the Denovillier's fascia can be incised and the entire posterior aspect of the prostate can be mobilized. In case of a nerve-sparing procedure an intrafacial technique for preparation has to start here.

Preparation of the pedicles/neurovascular bundles

The instruments used are:

- Right arm: cold scissors
- Left arm: bipolar forceps
- Assistant: suction, grasper, clipper (10 mm Hem-o-lok clips).

Starting at the prostate base the pedicles are mobilized using the cold scissors to avoid thermal injury. Clips are used tangentially to the prostate for hemostasis. Nerve sparing can be performed in a descending technique starting at this point. Care should be taken while using the clips to avoid clipping of the entire neurovascular bundles (NVBs). Alternatively, a combined descending and ascending technique is possible, as published by Patel et al.[7] After mobilizing the basal parts of the pedicles the preparation is continued from the apical and mid portion of the prostate mobilizing the NVBs.

Note: completely avoid any use of current during this process!

As the direction proceeds in a retrograde fashion the NVBs can be clearly identified and released off the prostate. Finally the pedicles can be clipped far away from the NVBs and sharp cut to release the prostate (Figure 16.9).

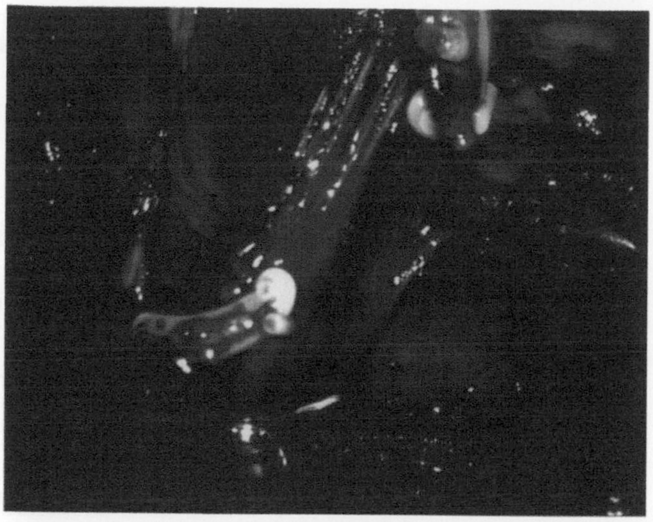

Figure 16.9 Intrafascial nerve sparing is performed by incision of the periprostatic fascia and mobilizing the entire NVB.

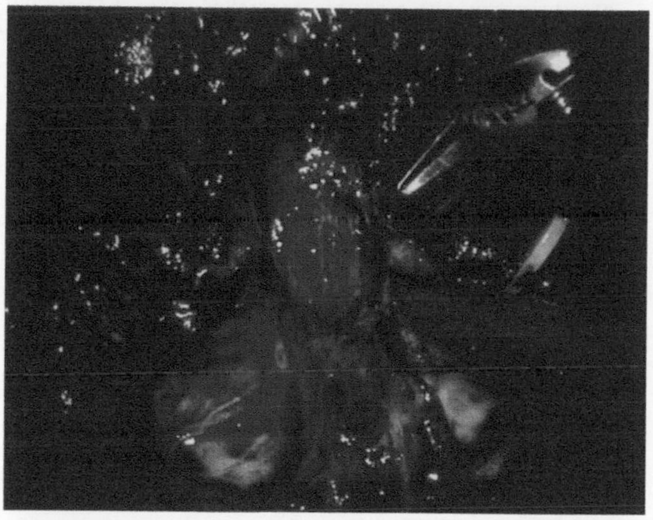

Figure 16.10 The apex has been mobilized creating a long urethral stump.

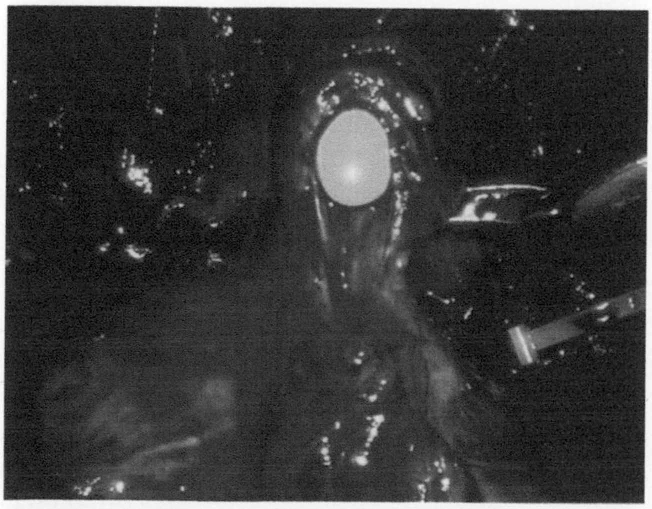

Figure 16.11 The urethra is incised at the apex under direct vision.

Apical resection

The instruments used are:

- Right arm: scissors
- Left arm: bipolar forceps
- Assistant: suction, grasper.

Incision has to be done cranially of the DVC ligation, keeping the suture intact. The urethra is identified and mobilized completely. If nerve sparing is performed, cold scissors should be used to divide the DVC and a long, thick urethral stump is created. The urethra is cut stepwise, making sure that the apex of the prostate is not affected (Figures 16.10–16.11).

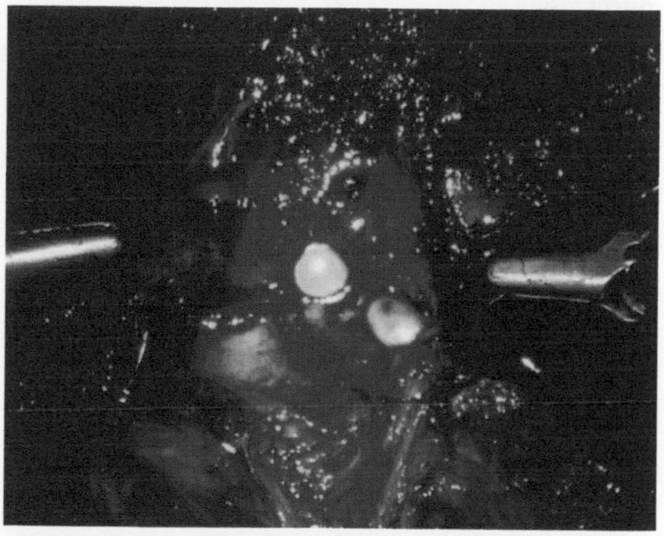

Figure 16.12 Posterior urethral anastomosis is performed with a running suture according to Van Velthoeven's technique.

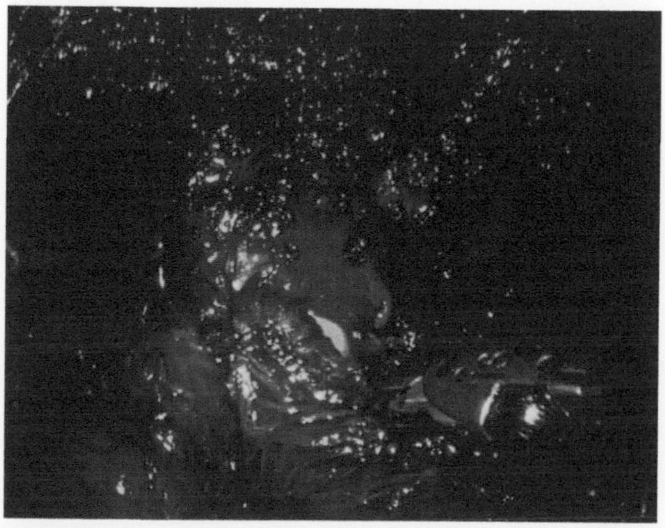

Figure 16.13 Completion of the anastomosis to the ventral aspect (left side finished).

Urethrovesical anastomosis

The instruments used are:

- Right/left arm: needle drivers
- Assistant: suction, grasper, scissors.

The anastomosis is performed by the Van Velthoefen technique,[9] using a 16 cm running suture of 3 × 0 PDS with RB-1 needles. After the first three to four dorsal stitches the bladder is carefully brought down to the urethra (Figures 16.12). An 18–20F Foley catheter is inserted and the suture is completed and tied at the 12 o'clock position (Figure 16.13). Saline irrigation is used to confirm that a water-tight anastomosis has been achieved, the specimen is harvested, and all trocars are removed under direct vision.

REFERENCES

1. Hance J, Aggarwal R, Undre S, Darzi A. Skills training in telerobotic surgery. Int J Med Robot 2005; 1(2): 7–12.
2. Horgan S, Benedetti E, Moser F. Robotically assisted donor nephrectomy for kidney transplantation. Am J Surg 2004; 188 (Suppl): 45S–51S.
3. Kaul S, Laungani R, Sarle R et al. Da Vinci-assisted robotic partial nephrectomy: technique and results at a mean of 15 months of follow-up. Eur Urol 2007; 51(1): 186–91.
4. Chammas MF, Hubert J, Patel VR. Robotically assisted laparoscopic pyeloplasty: a transatlantic comparison of techniques and outcomes. BJU Int 2007; 99: 1113–17.
5. Pruthi RS, Wallen EM. Robotic-assisted laparoscopic radical cystoprostatectomy. Eur Urol 2007 (in press).
6. Menon M, Tewari A, Peabody J. Vattikuti Institute prostatectomy: a technique of robotic radical prostatectomy for management of localized carcinoma of the prostate: experience of over 1100 cases. Urol Clin North Am 2004; 31: 701–7.
7. Patel VR, Shah KK, Thaly RK, Lavery H. Robotic-assisted laparoscopic radical prostatectomy: the Ohio State University technique. J Robotic Surgery 2007; 1: 51–9.
8. Abbou CC, Hoznek A, Salomon L et al. Laparoscopic radical prostatectomy with a remote controlled robot. J Urol 2001; 165: 1964–6.
9. Van Velthoeven RF, Ahlering TE, Peltier A et al. Technique of laparoscopic running urethrovesical anastomosis: the single knot method. Urology 2003; 61(4): 699–702.

CHAPTER 17

Intrafascial nerve-sparing endoscopic extraperitoneal radical prostatectomy (nsEERPE) – technique step by step

Jens-Uwe Stolzenburg, Robert Rabenalt, Minh Do, Anja Dietel, Alan McNeill, and Evangelos N Liatsikos

INDICATION

As there are no specific selection criteria or special contraindications for endoscopic extraperitoneal radical prostatectomy (EERPE), the indications are the same as for open radical retropubic prostatectomy (clinically localized prostate cancer – T1 and T2 tumors).

Surgical treatment of clinical stage T3 carcinoma remains controversial, and for some authors it remains a contraindication, mainly due to an increased risk of positive surgical margins, lymph node metastases, and a less favorable long-term outcome. Nevertheless, there have been no randomized clinical trials comparing treatment options and their respective long-term outcomes in these patients. The arguments in favor of surgical treatment of clinical T3 tumors are the potential for adjuvant external beam radiotherapy (e.g. intensity modulated radiotherapy) where there are positive margins, and the avoidance of complications associated with locally advanced disease (e.g. hematuria, retention due to clot formation, ureteral obstruction). According to the European Association of Urology Guidelines (2006 edition), surgery can be considered as a therapeutic option for patients with clinical T3 carcinoma of the prostate, but it should be remembered that EERPE for clinical T3 cancer requires considerable experience and should be avoided by beginners.

Accepted criteria for the performance of unilateral or bilateral nerve-sparing (ns)EERPE are the following. Preoperative erectile function sufficient for intercourse (a). Clinically organ confined prostate cancer (b). Patients with PSA < 10 ng/ml and Gleason sum < 7 are those often regarded as best candidates for a nerve-sparing procedure (c); however, patients with a less favorable profile (Gleason score 7 or PSA 10–20 ng/ml) may also be considered on an individual basis. Intraoperative frozen section may be helpful in this setting.

Contraindications for a nerve-sparing technique are the following. Gleason score 8–10 prostate cancer and/or PSA > 20 ng/ml (a). Tumor invasion within the neurovascular bundle (intraoperative frozen section) (b). Induration at the apex or posterolateral borders of the prostate (intraoperative decision) (c).

PREOPERATIVE SCHEDULE

We administer an enema on the evening before surgery and one early in the morning of the operative day. No further bowel preparation is necessary. Additional epidural anesthesia is not required. The risk of blood transfusion in our series is under 1%, therefore our patients are not advised to donate autologous blood. Broad-spectrum antibiotics are administered perioperatively.

Invasive intraoperative monitoring with a central line is not necessary and only two peripheral venous lines are placed. An arterial line is not usually necessary. Insertion of a nasogastric tube (moderate head down position, extraperitoneal access) is not needed. The body temperature of the patient is only measured when the operative period is extended due to an unexpected technical difficulty.

INSTRUMENTATION

- Standard laparoscopic tower: high-flow (carbon dioxide) insufflator, monitor, camera (Olympus Visera camera OTV-S7), light source CLV-S40, video laparoscope (EndoEye) – 0° optic 10 mm for VISERA control unit 'OTV-S7V-B' set, SonoSurg-Generator 'SonoSurg G2' (ultrasonic surgical system)

- Trocars: 1× Balloontrokar PDB 1000 (Tyco), 1× Hasson type optical trocar, 1× 12 mm trocar with reduction tube, and 3× 5.5 mm trocars
- Instruments (Olympus): 2× dissection forceps (HiQ+, 5 × 330 mm, straight), 1× grasping forceps (HiQ+, 5 × 330 mm), 1× grasping forceps (HiQ+, 5 × 330 mm, wave type), 1× laparoscopic Metzenbaum scissors, 1× SonoSurg scissors (5 mm), 1× bipolar forceps (HiQ+, Johann), Challenger Ti Clip Applicator (Aesculap) 1× 10 mm and 1× 5 mm, 2× needle holders, 1 endo-bag (Tyco).

TECHNIQUE OF nsEERPE STEP-BY-STEP

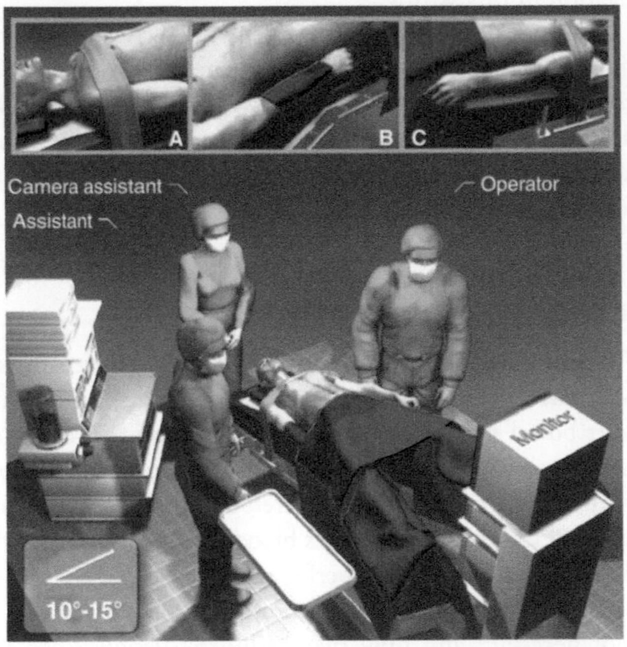

Figure 17.1 The patient is placed in a dorsal supine position (10° head down tilt) with legs slightly apart. The surgeon stands to the left of the patient with the assistant opposite, whilst the camera-holder stands at the head of the patient. All patients are supported with a chest belt (A). Both arms are protected, positioned on the body of the patient. The right arm is directly positioned at the body (in order to measure blood pressure) and with a sheet directly fixed using the weight of the patient (B). The left arm is positioned at a slight distance from the body (infusion arm) (C). Both legs are draped on the table as well, minimizing the risk of the patient's dislocation during the procedure. An 18Ch Foley catheter is inserted under sterile conditions.

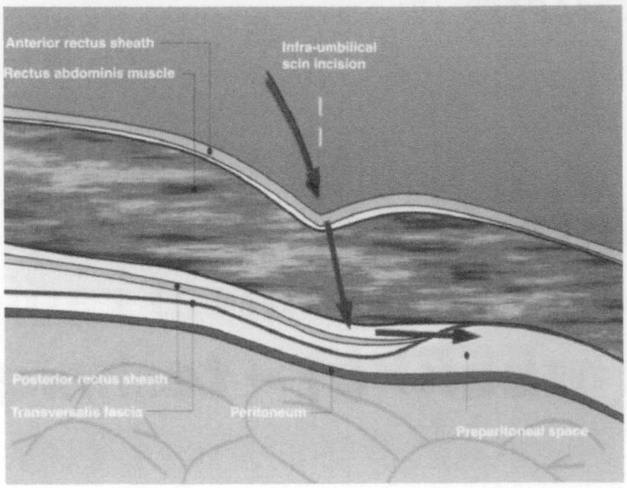

Figure 17.2 The first step is to create a preperitoneal space. An oblique 15 mm incision is made in the infra-umbilic crease to the right of the midline and carried down to the anterior rectus fascia. The anterior rectus fascia is horizontally incised, exposing the rectus muscle. The rectus muscle fibers are vertically separated by blunt dissection, exposing the posterior rectus fascia. The space posterior to the rectus muscle and anterior to the posterior rectus sheath is bluntly developed by finger dissection. Thereafter, a balloon trocar is introduced anterior to the posterior rectus sheath and inflated under direct visual control.

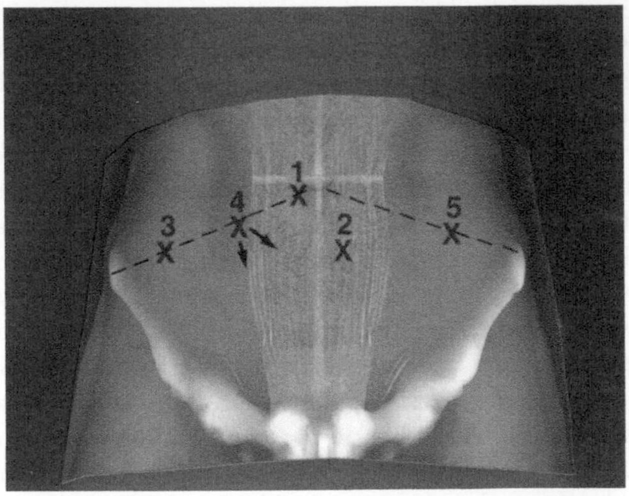

Figure 17.3 After removal of the balloon trocar an optical trocar (Hassan type) is introduced and fixed. CO_2 is insufflated to a pressure of 12 mmHg. The sequence and sites of trocar placement are shown: a 5 mm trocar, two finger-breadths left lateral to the midline (at a one-third to two-thirds ratio from the umbilicus to the public arch); a 5 mm trocar two finger-breadths medial to the right anterior superior iliac spine; a 5 mm trocar in the right pararectal line, taking care to avoid injury of the epigastric vessels by visual guidance during placement. The left preperitoneal space is now bluntly dissected from the right side. The final 12 mm trocar is placed approximately three finger-breadths medial to the left anterior superior iliac spine on a line towards the umbilicus.

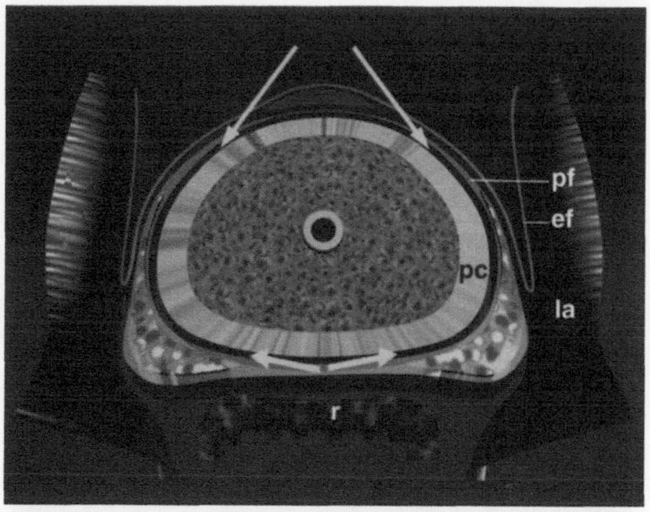

Figure 17.4 This figure illustrates the principles of intrafascial nerve-sparing radical prostatectomy. During 'standard' nerve-sparing prostatectomy the endopelvic fascia (ef) is incised and the neurovascular bundles (nvb) are spared posterolaterally between the endopelvic fascia and the periprostatic fascia (= interfascial technique). During intrafascial nerve-sparing endoscopic extraperitoneal prostatectomy we incise the endopelvic fascia only ventrally medial to the puboprostatic ligaments. Then, we dissect on the prostatic capsule (pc), freeing the prostate laterally from its thin surrounding fascia (pf, periprostatic fascia), which contains small vessels and nerves. The dorsal dissection plane is between Denonvilliers' fascia and the prostatic capsula. la, levator ani; r, rectum.

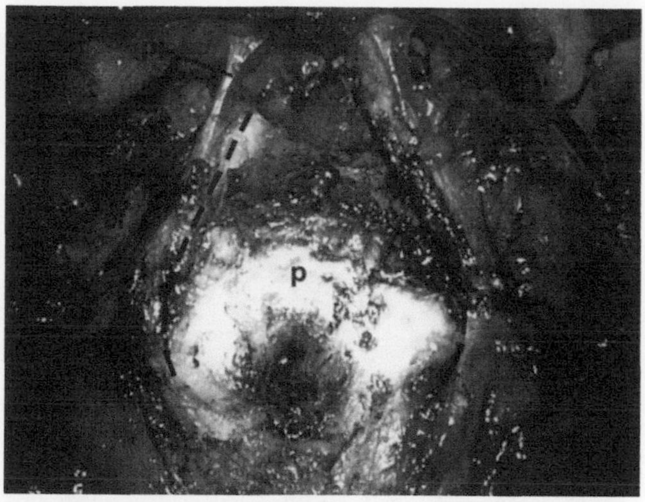

Figure 17.6 During intrafascial nsEERPE the endopelvic fascia (ef) is not incised at the beginning of the procedure as performed in 'wide excision' EERPE. Starting from the bladder neck (bn) a bilateral sharp incision of the superficial fascia overlaying the prostate (p) is performed distally toward the apex medial to the puboprostatic ligaments (pl) on both sides (see interrupted lines). The plane (see Figure 17.4) between the prostate and its thin overlaying fascia (intrafascial) is developed to guide further dissection later during the nerve-sparing procedure. When in the right plane a shiny surface of the prostate is visible that is easily dissected from the periprostatic fascia.

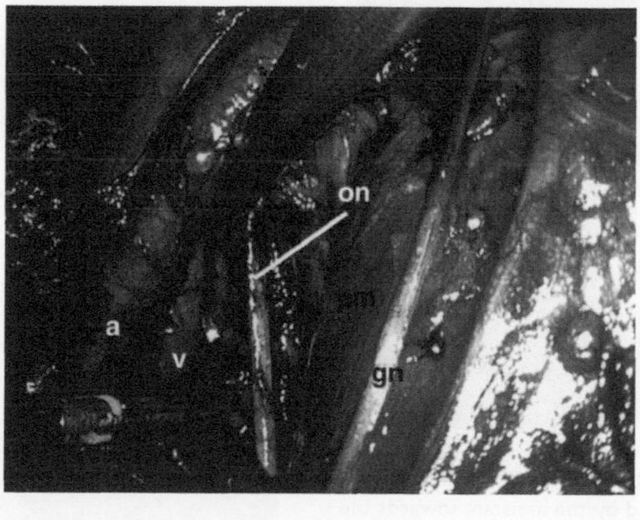

Figure 17.5 Pelvic lymph node dissection is performed in patients with PSA > 10 ng/ml and/or Gleason sum > 6. The lymphadenectomy is commenced on the left. The assistant retracts the lymph nodes whilst the surgeon dissects between the lymph node and the iliac vessels. The lymph vessels are identified, clipped, and cut with the aid of the SonoSurg device, and lymphatic tissue is meticulously dissected from the external iliac artery (a) and vein (v). Next the lymphatic tissue is dissected from the obturator fossa. The obturator nerve (on) is freed caudally to cranially. The figure shows the completely dissected external iliac artery, its adjacent psoas muscle (pm) and genitofemoral nerve (gn) (lateral border for the lymphadenectomy). The vessels are retracted medially and the entire obturator fossa is thus completely freed from its lymphatic tissue. Starting from the external iliac artery the dissection is continued in a caudo-cranial direction. The junction of the internal iliac with the external iliac artery marks the upper limit of the lymph node dissection.

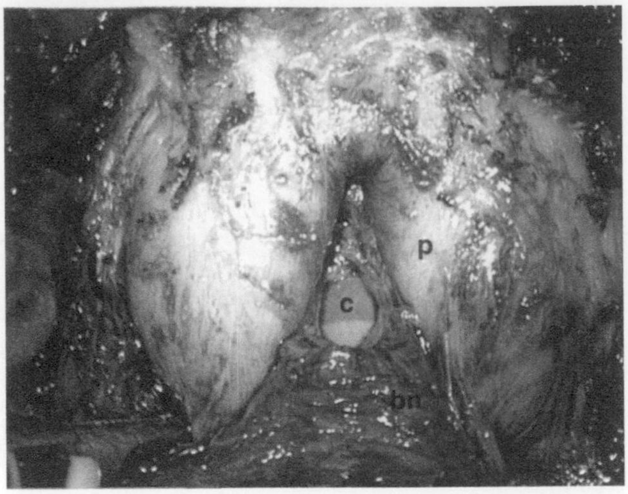

Figure 17.7 The next step of the procedure is the anterior bladder neck dissection. The surgeon and the assistant have to push the base of the developed bladder neck (bn) dorsally to better visualize the bladder neck. The previously created superficial incision is enlarged and deepened from 10 to 2 o'clock with the SonoSurg device to identify the longitudinal musculature of the bladder neck. The longitudinal musculature is only present around the urethra at the bladder neck, when it is incised the catheter (c) becomes visible. p, prostate.

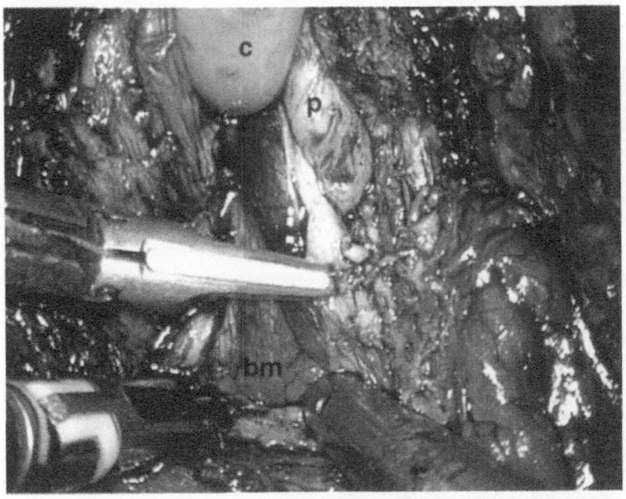

Figure 17.8 As soon as the urethra is incised at the 12 o'clock position the catheter (c) is retracted by the assistant towards the symphisis. Note that you should exert traction to the catheter with a clamp at the level of the external urethral meatus. The dissection is now continued laterally in the plane between bladder neck and prostate (p). The figure demonstrates the posterior bladder neck dissection. The dissection needs to follow a perpendicular plane to ensure access to the vas. It is important to avoid oblique dissection as this will lead to dissection into the prostate. The posterior bladder neck must first be completely divided between the 5 and 7 o'clock position. bm, bladder mucosa.

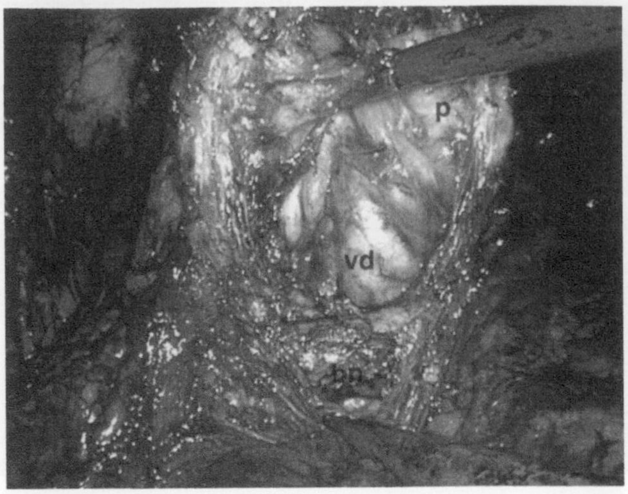

Figure 17.9 The key anatomic landmarks during posterior bladder neck (bn) dissection are the ampullary portions of the vasa deferentia (vd). When these structures have been identified the posterior bladder neck dissection is extended laterally in both directions. Both vasa are divided with the SonoSurg device, then the seminal vesicles are freed in turn as the assistant retracts the ipsilateral vas contralaterally and cranially with the forceps on the right hand, and with the suction on the left hand the assistant pushes the bladder down. This provides good visualization to the seminal vesicle. The surgeon can now proceed to dissect the seminal vesicle step by step from its surrounding structures. p, prostate.

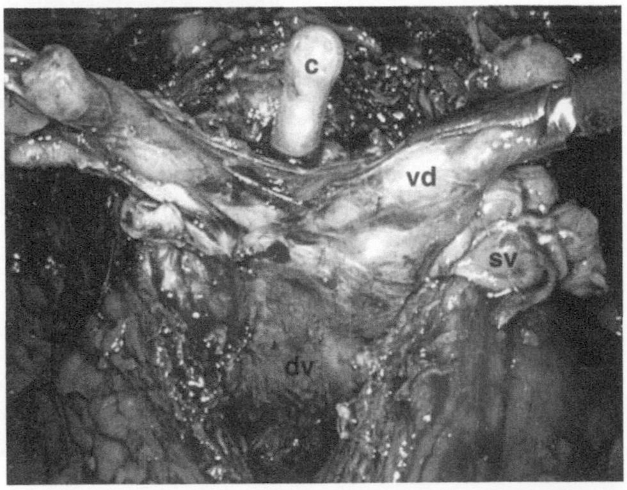

Figure 17.10 Once dissection of the seminal vesicles (sv) is complete the assistant holds the right ampulla and the right seminal vesicle, the surgeon has the left ampulla and the left seminal vesicle in a craniolateral direction. With this maneuver an 'anatomical window' is developed, which reaches from the dorsal aspect of the prostate to the prostatic pedicles. Between these structures the posterior layer of Denonvillier's fascia (dv) is clearly seen. c, catheter; vd, vas deferens.

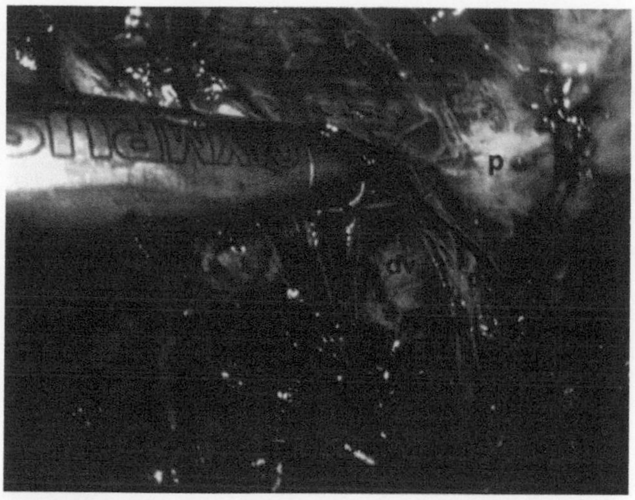

Figure 17.11 In contrast to the 'standard' nerve-sparing technique (= interfascial) we do not incise the Denonvillier's fascia (dv) in intrafascial nsEERPE. Therefore, the prerectal fatty tissue does not become visible. The appropriate plane is found by stripping Denonvillier's fascia from the prostatic capsule. This maneuver is performed entirely by blunt dissection. Complete mobilization of Denonvillier's fascia and all adherent tissue is performed by staying close to the posterior surface of the prostatic capsule to gain medial access to the prostatic pedicle and neurovascular bundles. bl, bladder; p, prostate.

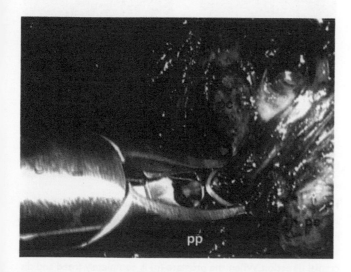

Figure 17.12 Next follows dissection of the prostatic pedicle (pp). At this point of the procedure we have created two safe planes. Medially as well as laterally the 'shining' surface of the prostatic capsule (pc) may be clearly seen. During dissection of the left prostatic pedicle, the assistant retracts the partially mobilized prostate to the right side, and vice versa. The prostatic pedicle and small vessels have to be clipped and divided between endo-clips.

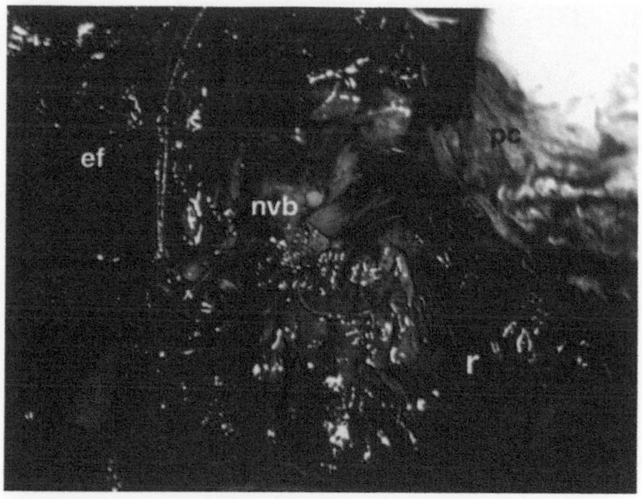

Figure 17.13 Traction is applied to the seminal vesicles by pulling each out of the pelvis in a contralateral direction, whilst the ipsilateral neurovascular bundles (nvb) are carefully freed. The main parts of the neurovascular bundles are attached to the dorsolateral surface of the prostate. Using clips and 'cold' scissors, the neurovascular bundles are completely separated from the prostate during prostatic pedicle dissection. It is advisable to proceed with the clipping and cutting in small steps. The SonoSurg device is only used as a blunt dissecting tool during this part of the procedure. pc, prostatic capsule; ef, endopelvic fascia; r, rectum.

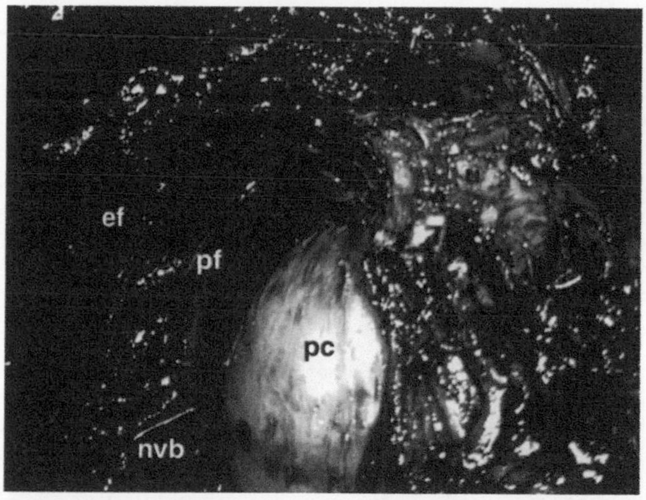

Figure 17.14 When the prostate has been mobilized dorsally and laterally it is pushed to the contralateral side of the pelvis to provide good access to the apex and the urethra. The mobilized puboprostatic ligaments and the remaining puboprostatic fascia (pf) on the lateral surface of the prostate are now completely detached from the urethra (u) and the apex. After full mobilization the Santorini plexus is clearly visualized from the lateral aspect. A 2-0 Polysorb GS-22 needle (slightly straightened) is then used and guided from left to right in the plane below the dorsal venous complex, and the plexus is thus ligated. During this step the assistant pushes the prostate dorsocranially to elongate the urethra. pc, prostatic capsule; ef, endopelvic fascia; nvb, neurovascular bundles.

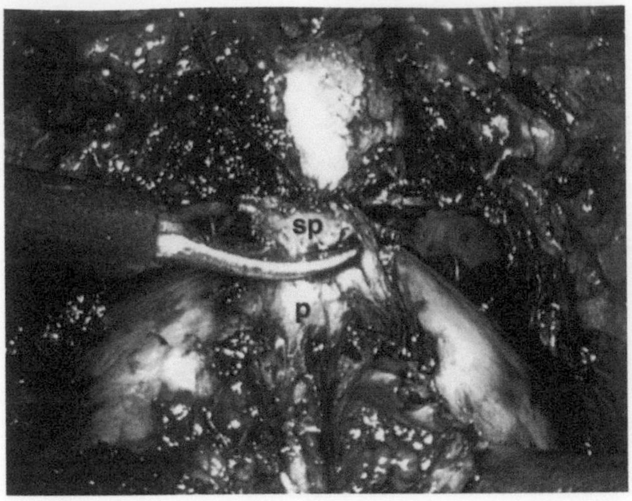

Figure 17.15 Apical dissection is then undertaken using Metzenbaum scissors respecting the shape of the prostate (p) and the course of the external sphincter, which overlaps the prostate ventrally, to protect as many striated muscle fibers of the external sphincter as possible. For this reason dissection is not perpendicular, as a strictly perpendicular dissection would leave residual prostatic tissue dorsally and could generate positive margins. The actual apical dissection is a three-step procedure, which starts with dissection of the Santorini plexus (sp). This is performed lateral to medial, from left to right, until full dissection is completed.

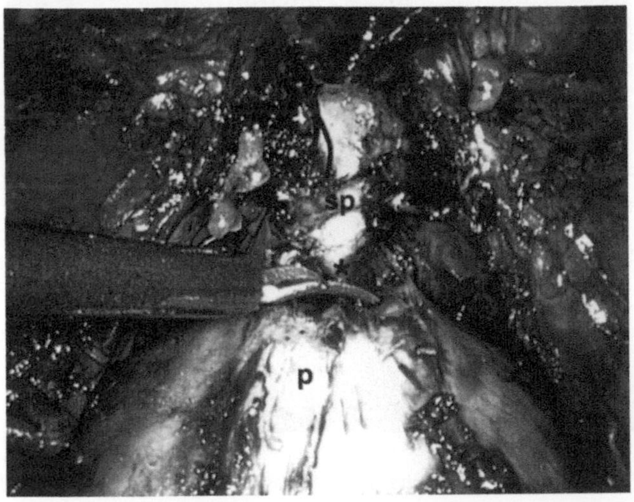

Figure 17.16 After the Santorini plexus (sp) has been dissected, the border between the prostate (p) and the urethra (external sphincter, the striated part is marked with an asterisk) is found lateral at 9 and 3 o'clock positions. The dissection of the junction between urethral sphincter (external sphincter) and prostate is the second step of the apical dissection. The dissection converges medially from both sides. For optimal access the prostate should be pushed dorsocranially by the assistant. Ensuring that the catheter is inserted within the urethra and visible at the proximal prostatic end facilitates apical dissection.

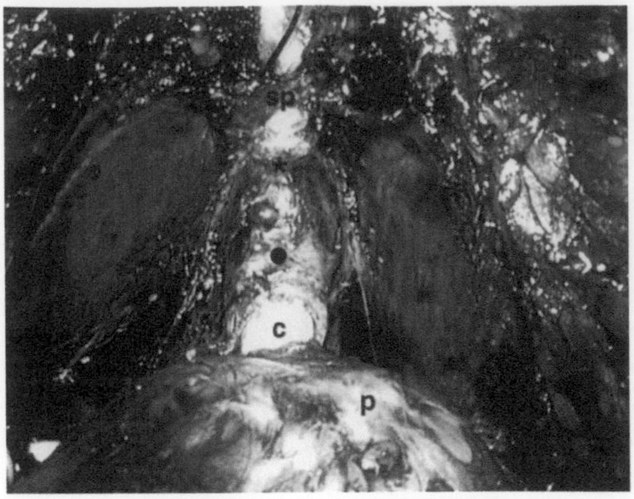

Figure 17.17 The third step of apical dissection is the dissection of the inner smooth muscular layer of the urethra (indicated by a black dot). By pushing the prostate craniocaudally a longer segment of the smooth urethra is achieved. Dissection of the anterior urethra is then performed proximally very close to the prostate (p) to preserve as long a length of urethra as possible. As soon as the urethral catheter (c) becomes visible the assistant retracts the catheter towards the symphisis. Dissection of the posterior urethra is then performed distal to the veru montanum. sp, Santorini plexus. The asterisk indicates the striated part of the external sphincter.

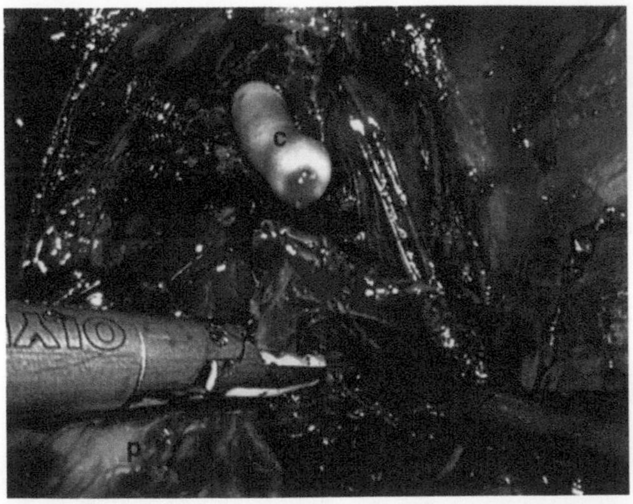

Figure 17.18 The final detachment of the posterior urethra (u) is performed dorsolaterally and from anterolaterally to avoid any injury to the neurovascular bundles (nvb) and the rectum. The assistant retracts the seminal vesicle contralaterally out of the pelvis in a cranial direction. When the prostate (p) is completely freed and dissected from its surrounding structures, it is placed in an endoscopic bag. In cases where there is suspicion of a positive margin the specimen can be immediately retracted through the 12 mm trocar site, by enlargement of the skin and fascial incision. The suspicious margin of the specimen should be marked with color and sent for frozen section. After specimen extraction the fascia is sutured and the trocar repositioned to continue with the anastomosis. c, catheter.

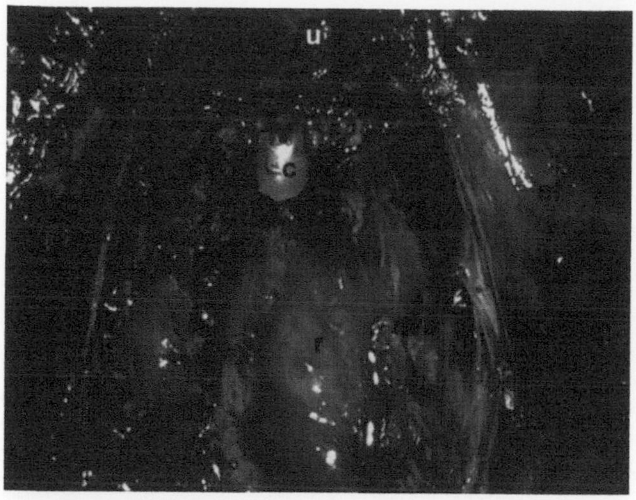

Figure 17.19 Intraoperative view of the pelvis after complete removal of the prostate following a bilateral nerve-sparing prostatectomy. The intrafacial dissection technique offers maximum protection to the neurovascular bundles (nvb), leaving not only the neurovascular bundles intact but also the puboprostatic ligaments (pl), the endopelvic fascia (ef), and the periprostatic fascia. When there is minor bleeding from the neurovascular bundle (surface hemorrhage and venous oozing), we recommend the use of TachoSil® (NYCOMED Austria GmbH). Coagulation is absolutely forbidden. Arterial bleeding will not be stopped by any hemostatic agent and must be controlled using clips. c, catheter; r, rectum; u, urethra.

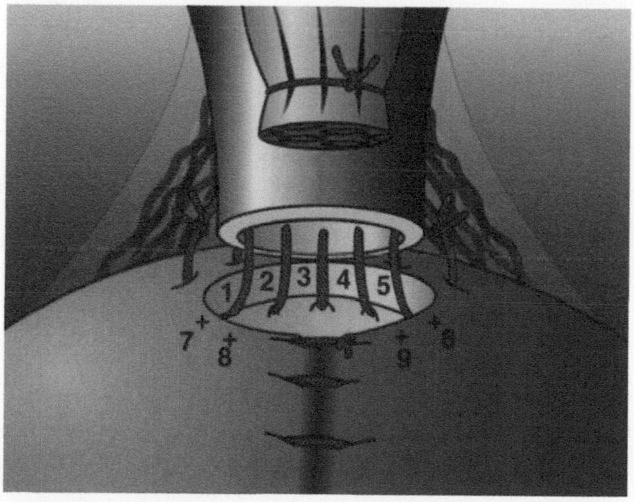

Figure 17.20 The urethra–vesical anastomosis is then performed with a 2-0 Polysorb on a GU-46 needle (alternative: UR-6 needle, 2-0 Vicryl). Depending on the size of the bladder neck, eight or nine sutures are necessary for a water-tight anastomosis. The sequence of stitches is shown. The stitch is always passed through the bladder neck first, 'outside-in', and then 'inside-out' at the urethra. In this way the sutures are always tied extraluminally. The first stitch starts at the 8 o'clock position. In case of widely open bladder neck, bladder neck closure (ventrally) should be performed before the final two anastomotic sutures at 11 and 1 o'clock positions. When commencing the anastomosis the Trendelenburg position is reduced to the minimum required.

POSTOPERATIVE SCHEDULE

The drain is removed 24–48 hours after the procedure. If the postoperative urine output through the urethral catheter is less than the output of the drain for more than 48 hours, then reintervention and reformation of the anastomosis should be carried out.

We routinely perform a cystogram before catheter removal. Provided that there is no leak, the catheter can be removed on the fifth or sixth postoperative day. Earlier catheter removal may be associated with acute urinary retention. If the cystogram shows a minor leak a further period of catheterization is required (3–7 days). An additional cystogram should be performed before catheter removal. If the leak persists longer catheterization time is deemed necessary. In all patients where we have observed a minor leak on the cystogram, there was no urine output from the drain. Antibiotic administration is necessary.

When there is a major leak, bilateral ureteric mono J catheters should be inserted to try and keep the bladder and anastomosis as 'dry' as possible. The mono J catheters should be fixed to the catheter carefully (suture) and should remain in place for 10–14 days. A cystogram should be performed before their removal.

CHAPTER 18

Laparoscopic radical prostatectomy – transperitoneal approach

Serdar Deger

INDICATION

Patients with localized histologically proven prostate cancer are candidates for laparoscopic radical prostatectomy (LRP). There is no specific indication for the transperitoneal approach

PREOPERATIVE SCHEDULE

- Diet: Patients have a normal breakfast in the morning, soup for lunch, and only fluid in the evening.
- Bowel preparation: No specific bowel preparation is necessary. Two rectal enemas are administered in the evening.
- Antibiotics: Third-generation cephalosporin and metronidazole as a single shot during surgery.

INSTRUMENTATION

- Mandantory:
  - 0° optic
  - Scissors with monopolar energy
  - Forceps with bipolar energy
  - Needle holder
- Optional:
  - Harmonic scalpel
  - Clip applicator
- Sutures:
  - CT-1 needle 0 vicryl
  - UR-6 needle 2×0 vicryl or 2-3×0 vicryl
- Trocars:
  - One 10 mm trocar for the scope
  - One 10 mm trocar as working trocar to introduce and remove needles or retracting devices
  - Three 5 mm working trocars.

STEP-BY-STEP OPERATIVE TECHNIQUE

The positioning of the patient, surgeons, and nurse is shown in Figure 18.1. The patient is placed supine with arms at the sides and secured with belts on the chest and thighs. (Figure 18.2). Following the establishment of a pneumoperitoneum of 15 mm Hg using Veress canula or minilaparatomy, five trocars can be positioned as shown in Figure 18.3.

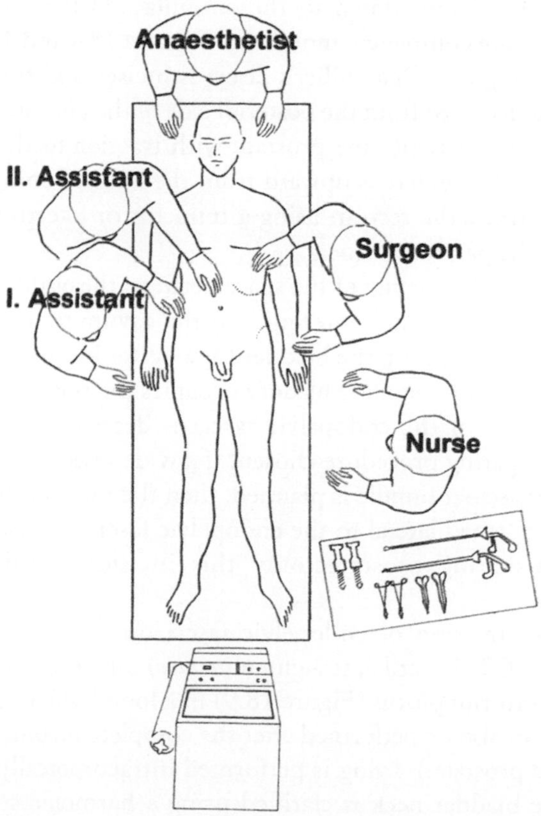

Figure 18.1 Positions of the patient, surgeons, and nurse in the operation room.

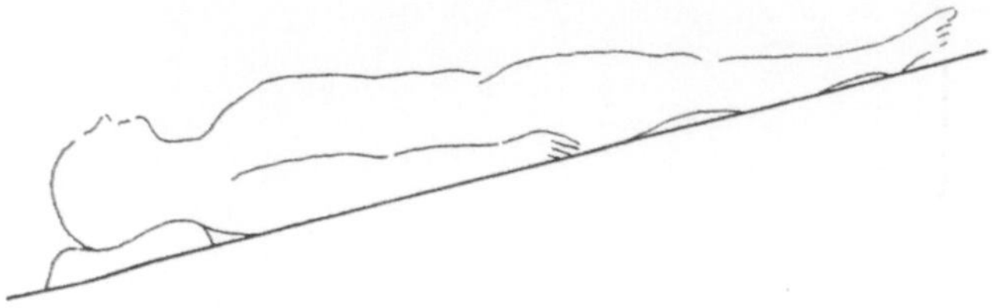

Figure 18.2 Position of the patient on the operation table.

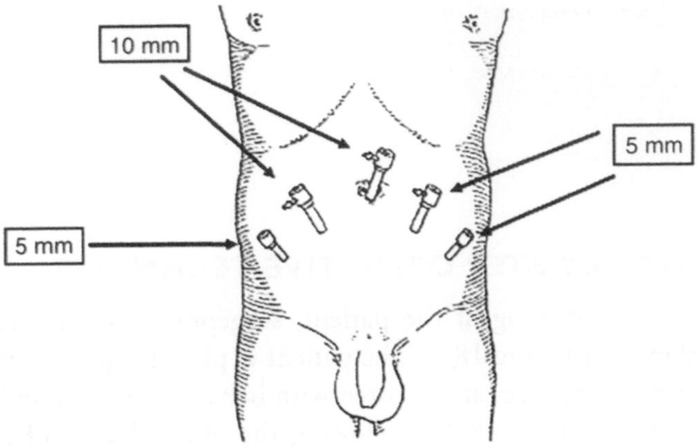

Figure 18.3 Positioning of five trocars.

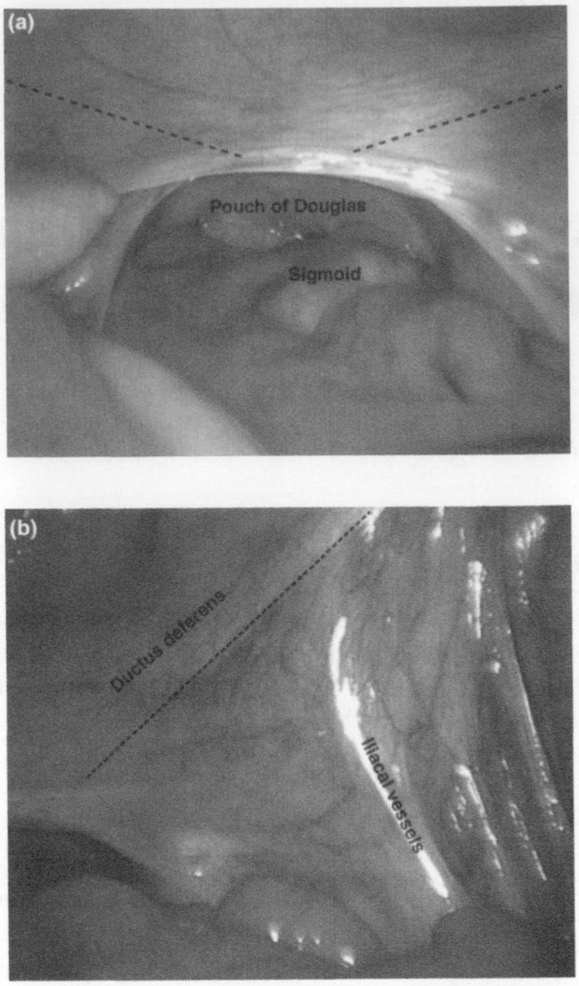

Figure 18.4 View and incision line in the pouch of Douglas (optional step) to reach the seminal vesicles.

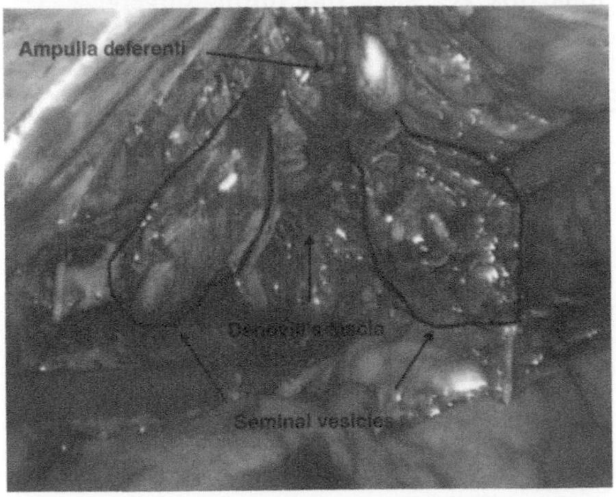

Figure 18.5 Complete mobilization of seminal vesicles.

After incision of the peritoneum in the pouch of Douglas the vas deferens down to the ampulla and the seminal vesicles are completely mobilized (Figures 18.4 and 18.5). Following this Denovillier's fascia is incised and the rectum is dissected from the posterior side of the prostate. The assistant can rotate the prostate with traction to the isolated ductus deferens upward from the lateral 5 mm port and retracts the rectum using a retractor or forceps from the right pararectal trocar.

As regards opening of the space between the bladder and abdominal wall and entering into the cavum rezii, it can be helpful to fill up the bladder for a better identification, but otherwise the filled bladder occupies the small pelvis.

Incision of the endopelvic fascia is dependent on the nerve-sparing procedure chosen. If a wide resection of the neurovascular bundle is planned, then the incision should be performed lateral to the endopelvic fascia. In case of a nerve-sparing prostatectomy this incision should be medial.

After incision of endopelvic fascia on both sides the suture (CT-1 vycril 0, straighten *in vitro*) can be put around the Santorini plexus (Figure 18.9) in a loop fashion. (This step can also be performed after the complete mobilization of the prostate.) Tying is performed intracorporeally.

The bladder neck is clarified using a harmonic scalpel and/or bipolar forceps with scissors (Figure 18.10). It is recommended that the bladder preparation is started medially and that the bladder is put under tension to identify layers easily. The muscular structures of the bladder neck can be clarified with stump dissection.

After opening the anterior wall of the bladder neck, the bladder catheter can be identified and put under traction from the lateral 5 mm port by the assistant, the bladder

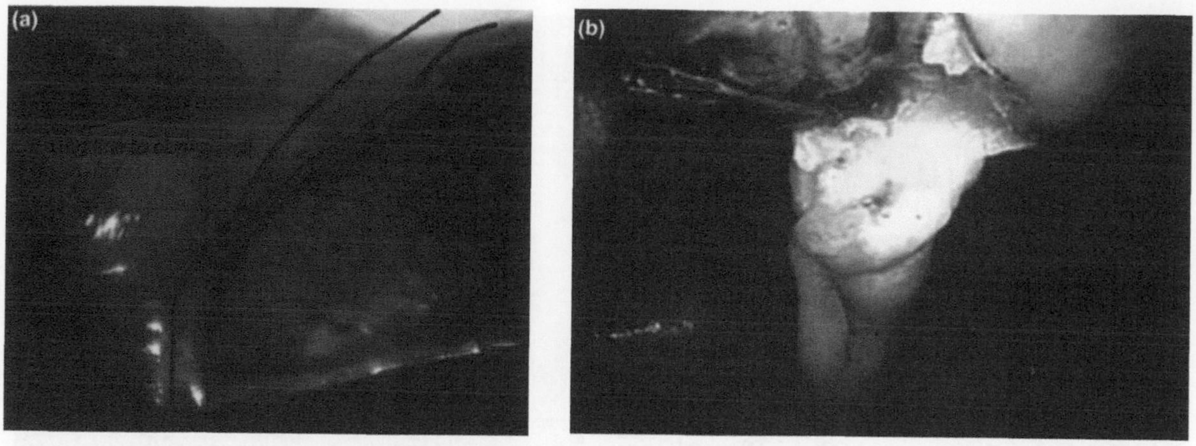

Figure 18.6 Incision line of obliterated ligament.

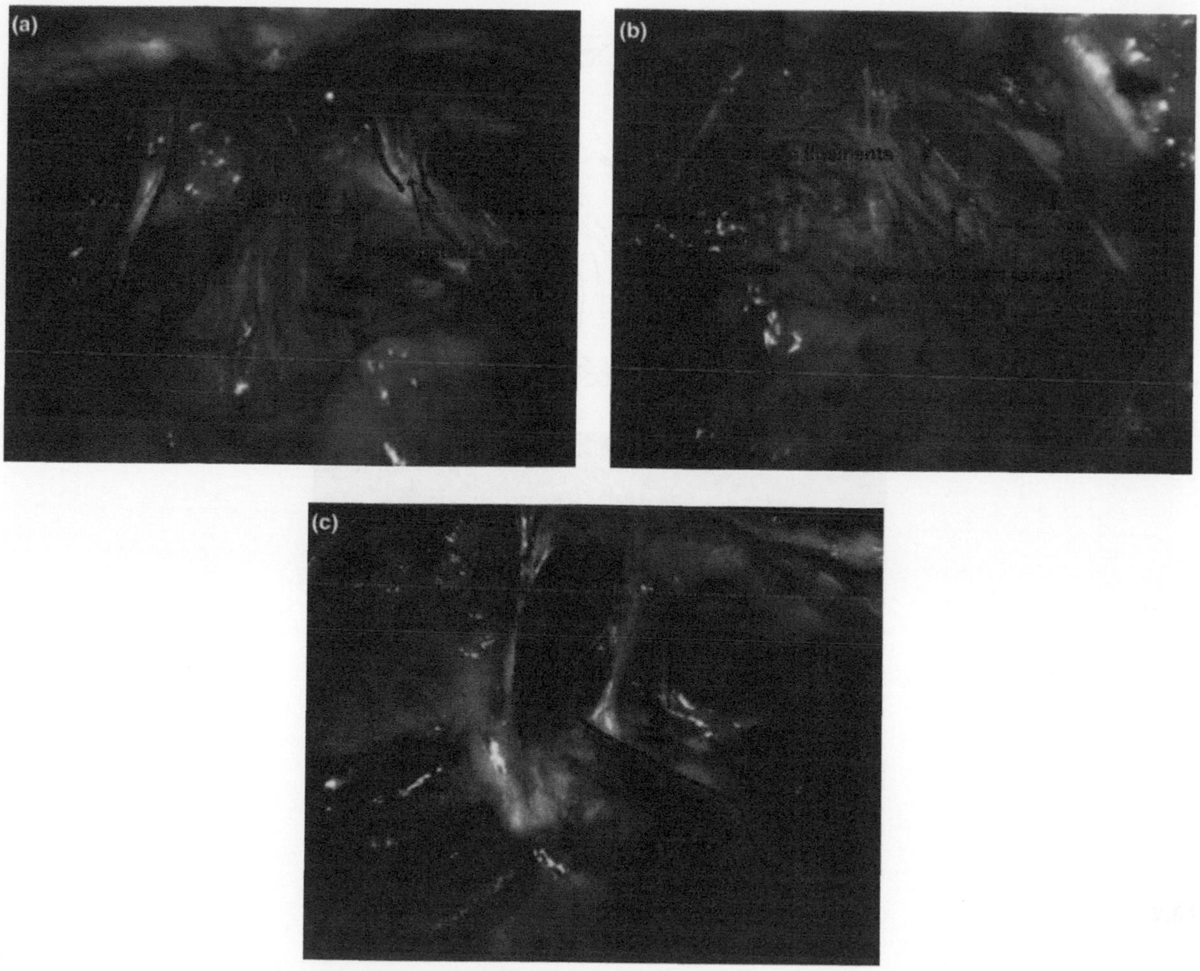

Figure 18.7 (a, b) View of the public arc. (c) Incision of endopelvic fascia.

can be retracted with a retractor or forceps from the medial 10 mm port by the assistant.

After dividing the posterior wall of the bladder neck, the seminal vesicles and ductus deferens can be extracted (Figure 18.11).

Seminal vesicles are put under tension by the surgeon or assistant to reach prostatic pedicles. In the non-nerve sparing LRP the pedicles can be divided using clips, monopolar or bipolar cautery, or harmonic scalpel (Figure 18.12).

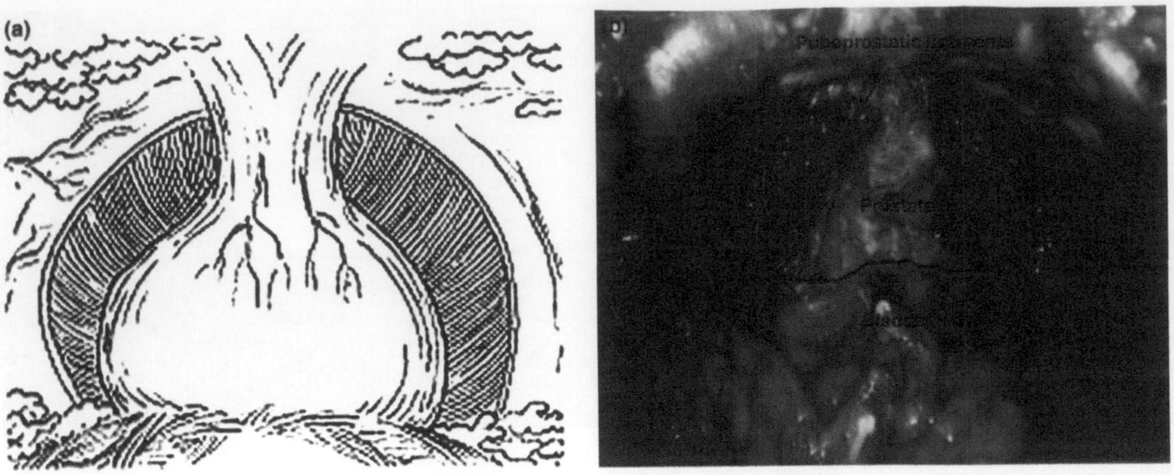

Figure 18.8

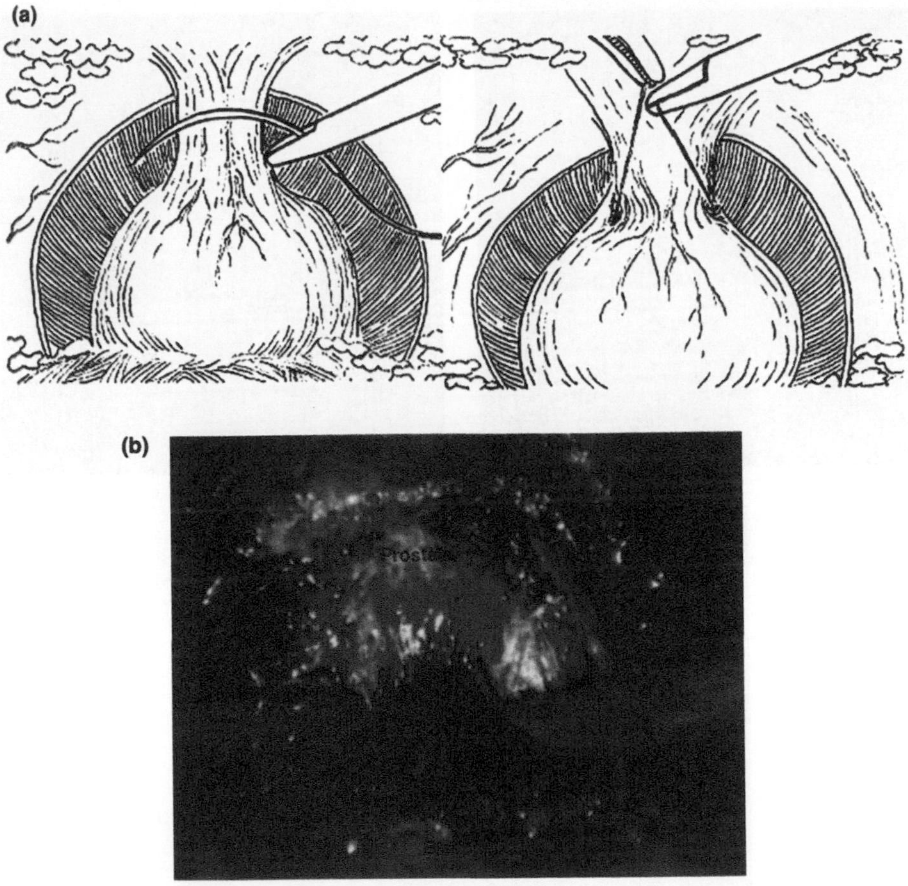

Figure 18.9

In a nerve-sparing procedure, the prostatic capsula can be incised and the neurovascular bundle (NVB) can be spared using sharp dissection. In the case of bleedings, 4×0 vicryl with an RB-1 needle can be used for stitching or clips can be applied. Coagulation should be avoided.

Following the complete mobilization of the prostate, the rectum can be checked by bringing water into the small pelvis and applying air through a tube into the rectum. Bubbles come to the surface when a rectal lesion is present.

Anastomosis can be carried out as interrupted sutures or as a running suture. A double-armed suture for running suture can ease the anastomosis. The bladder catheter should pass the posterior wall of the anastomosis

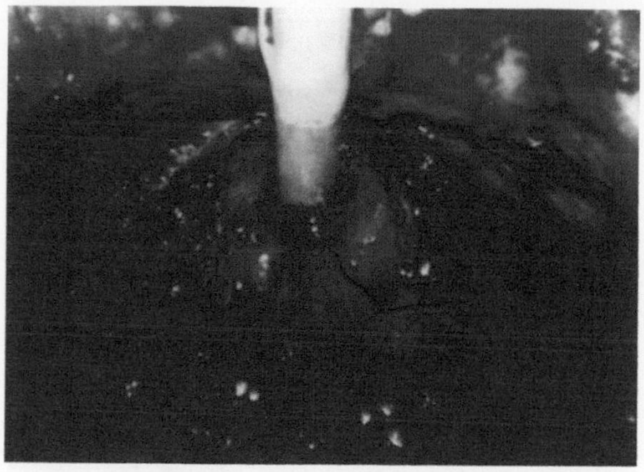

Figure 18.10 Retraction on the bladder catheter and bladder neck.

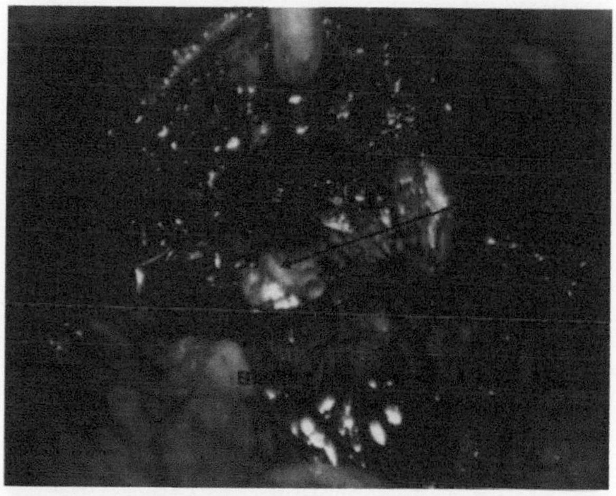

Figure 18.11 Retraction of the seminal vesicle.

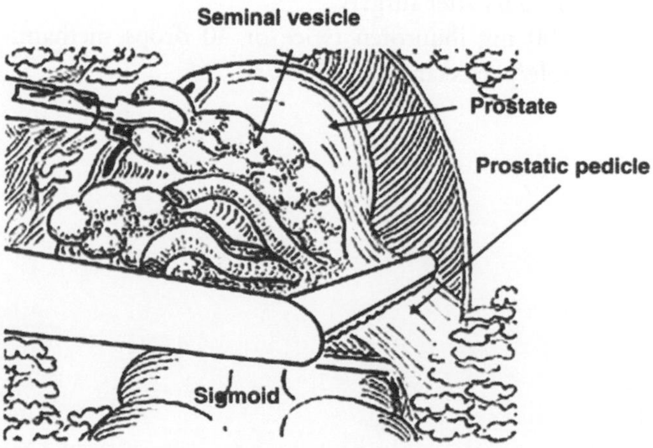

Figure 18.12 Division of prostatic pedicle.

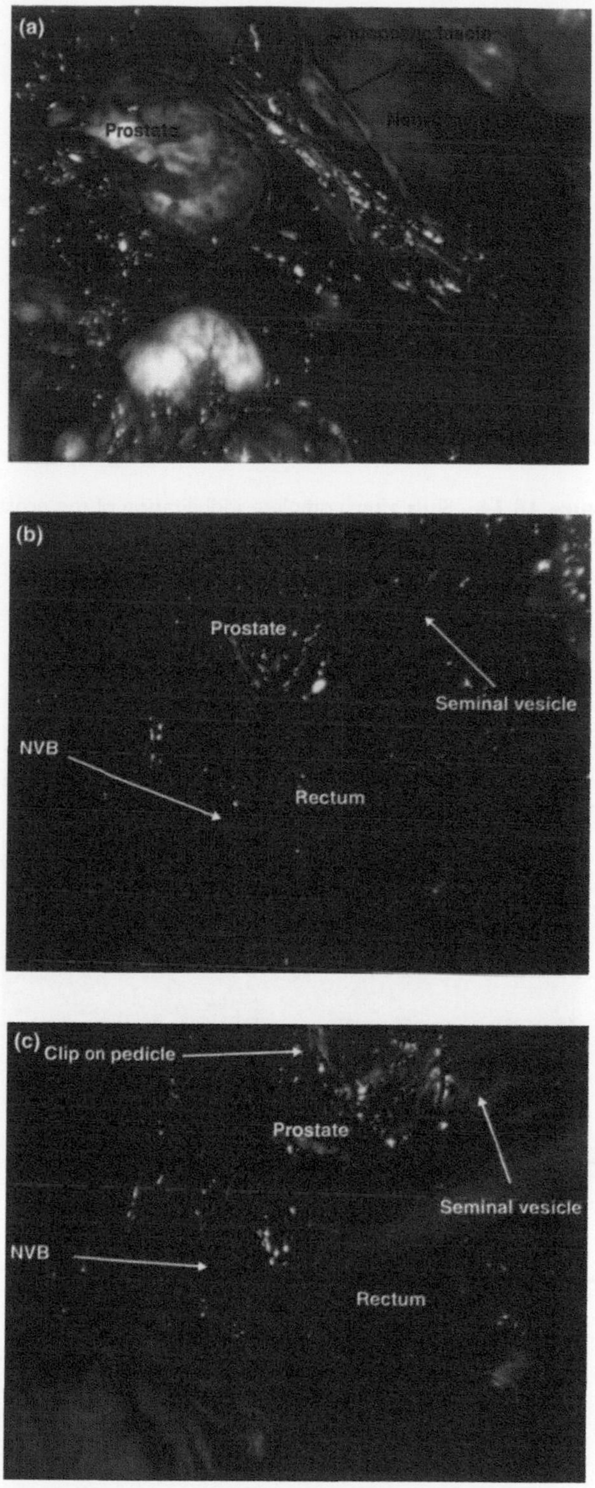

Figure 18.13 Exposure of the NVB.

without problems. The two pararectal ports (10 and 5 mm) can be used for anastomosis. A UR-6 needle is recommended.

After completion of the anastomosis the water-tightness must be checked by administering 200 ml of saline into the bladder via a Foley catheter.

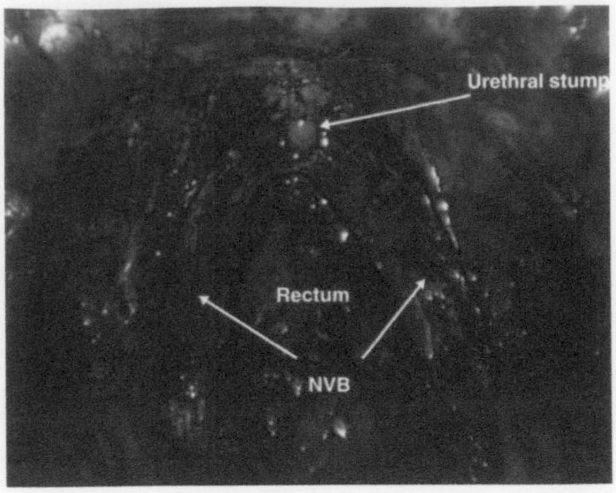

Figure 18.14 Situs after complete mobilization of the prostate in the nerve-sparing technique.

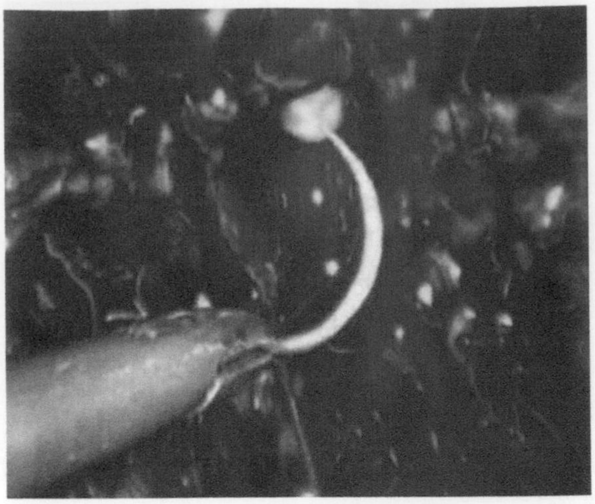

Figure 18.16 Passing the posterior wall of the urethra.

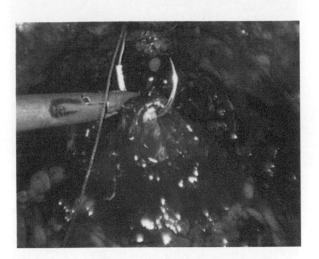

Figure 18.15 Passing the posterior wall of the bladder.

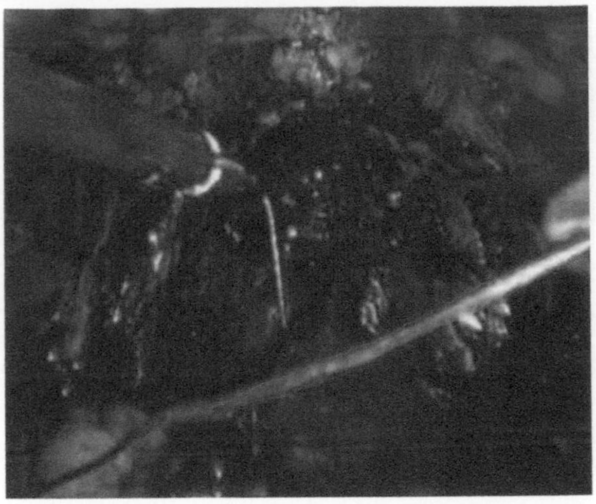

Figure 18.17 Tying is performed intracorporeally.

POSTOPERATIVE SCHEDULE

- Diet:
  Fluid intake 2 hours after surgery
  Yoghurt 4 hours after surgery
  Mobilization in the evening
  Next morning normal diet can be given
- Pain medication:
  1.5 g methamizole or 1 g paracetamol every 6 hours after surgery
  800 mg ibuprofen twice or 40 drops methamizole/paracetamol if necessary.

CHAPTER 19

Radical cystectomy in the male patient

Franco Gaboardi, Stefano Galli, Joannes Goumas, and Andrea Gregori

INTRODUCTION

Radical cystectomy remains the gold standard for invasive bladder cancer and the open technique with urinary diversion is the most common procedure. The laparoscopic technique is a minimally invasive treatment and an increasing number of authors have reported their initial experience.[1–8] However, the numbers in the series are limited, the follow-up periods are short, and various procedures have been described concerning radical cystectomy and urinary diversions.[7,9,10]

This chapter describes our technique[5,8] of laparoscopic radical cystectomy in males with ileal neobladder, named MILaN (Minimally Invasive Laparoscopic Neobladder).

LAPAROSCOPIC RADICAL CYSTOPROSTATECTOMY: STEP BY STEP

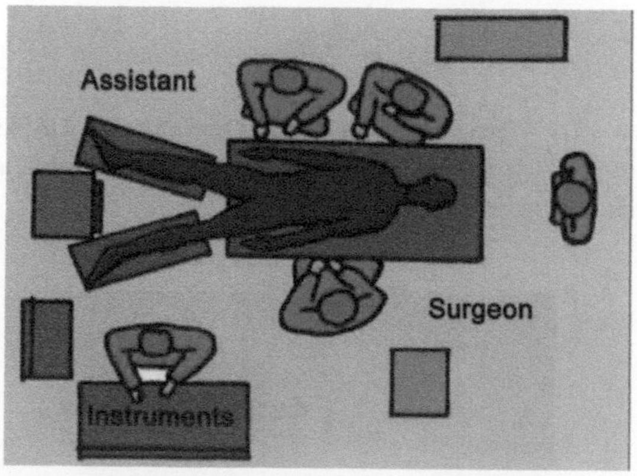

Figure 19.1 The positioning of the patient and personnel in the operating room.

Patient preparation

The bowel is prepared by oral administration of 2 litres of electrolyte lavage. Antibiostic prophylaxis and low-molecular-weight heparin are administered preoperatively.

The patient is placed in the supine position with the legs apart and the table is set in moderate Trendelenburg position. The surgeon is on the left side of the table with the first assistant in front and the second assistant (for the laparoscope) on the right of the first assistant. The nurse is on the left of the surgeon (Figure 19.1). The anesthetist is at the patient's head. The positions of the ports are shown in Figure 19.2.

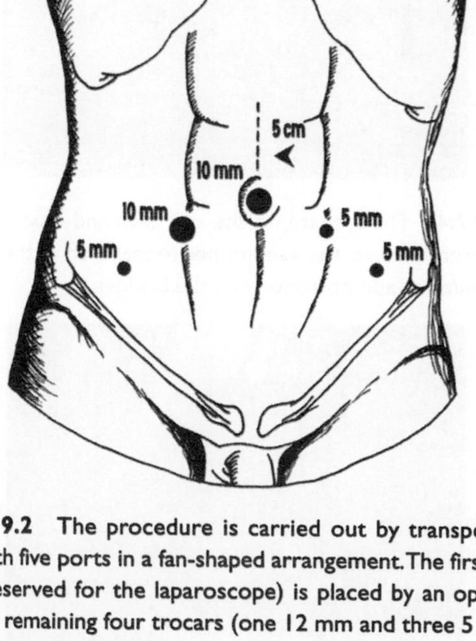

Figure 19.2 The procedure is carried out by transperitoneal access with five ports in a fan-shaped arrangement.The first 12 mm trocar (reserved for the laparoscope) is placed by an open technique, the remaining four trocars (one 12 mm and three 5 mm) are under endoscopic control.

Dissection of the vasa, seminal vesicles and Denonvillier's fascia incision

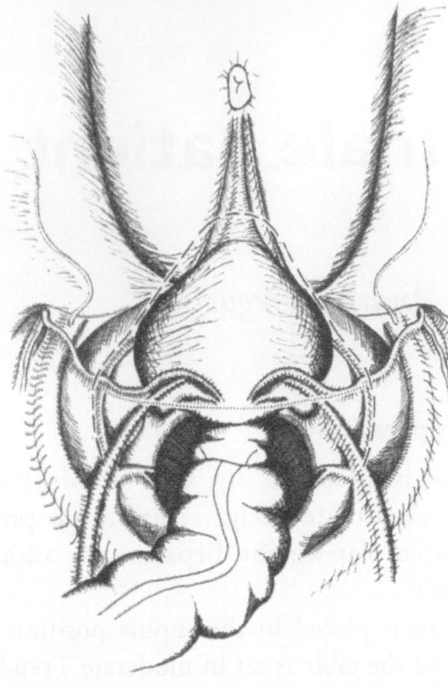

Figure 19.3 The first incision is at the level of the second peritoneal arch (dotted line).

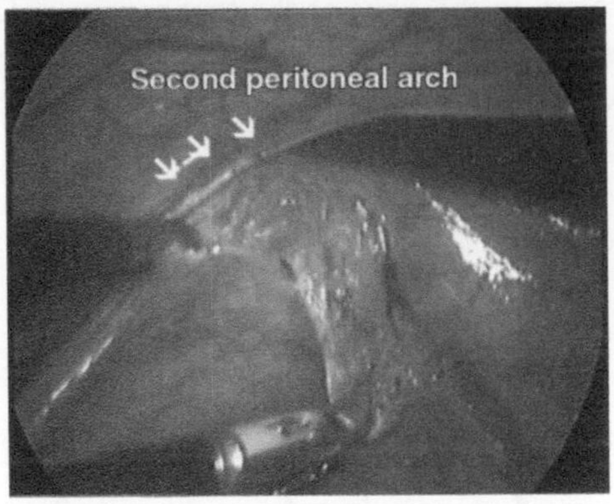

Figure 19.4 The first step is the approach and dissection of the vasa deferentia up to the second peritoneal arch in the pouch of Douglas inferior and posteriorly to the bladder.

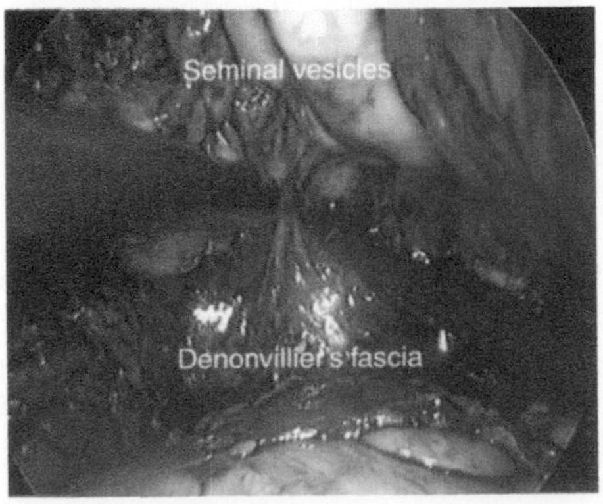

Figure 19.5 The seminal vesicles are isolated and maintained 'en bloc' with the bladder. The vasa and the seminal vesicles are retracted up to expose Denonvillier's fascia, which is incised horizontally.

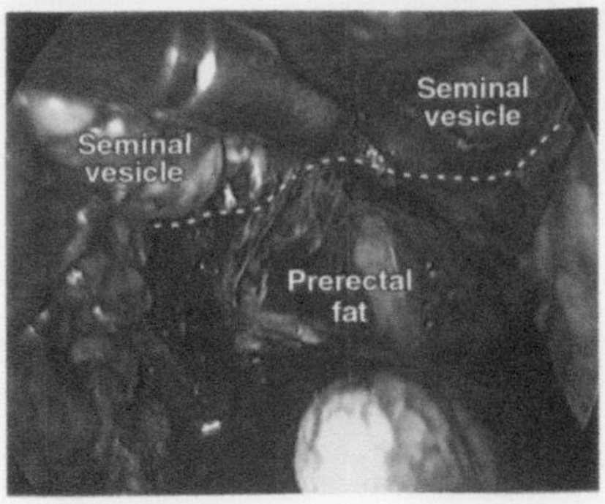

Figure 19.6 The incision permits the exposure of the prerectal fat and the anterior surface of the rectum is prepared up to the prostatic apex. A tunnel is created between the rectum and prostate and the vesical and prostatic pedicles appear like two tracks confluently to the prostatic apex.

Dissection of ureters

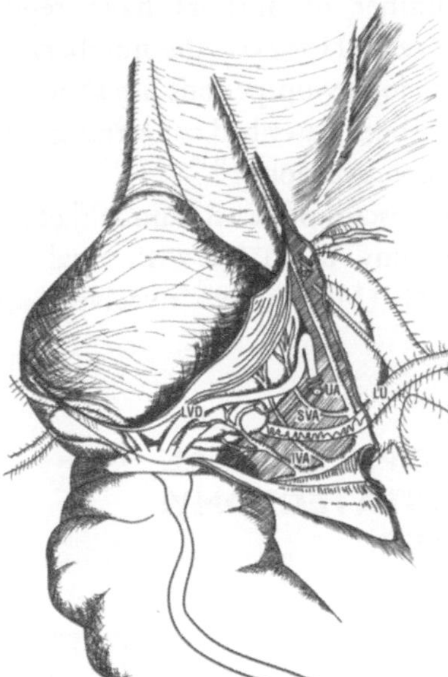

Figure 19.7 Dissection of ureter. LU, left ureter; UA, umbilical artery; IVA, inferior vesical artery; SVA, superior vesical artery; LVD, left vasa deferens.

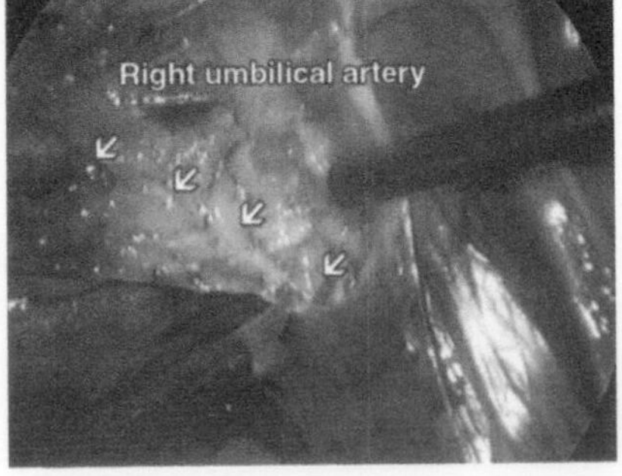

Figure 19.8 The right umbilical artery is identified and the peritoneum is incised just laterally to it.

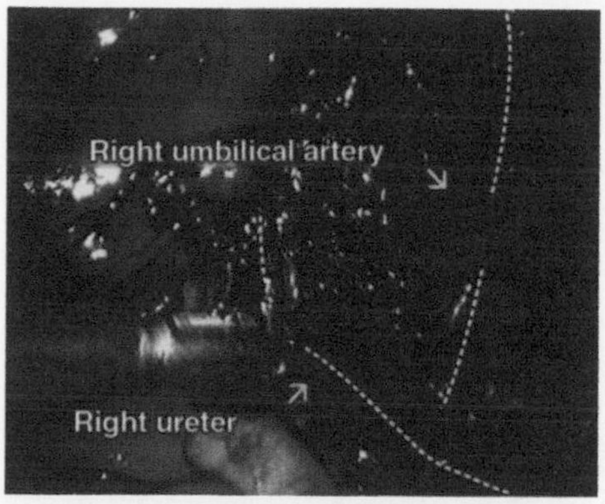

Figure 19.9 The right umbilical artery is isolated up to the deep iliac artery and the ureter is detected just medially to the origin of the umbilical artery.

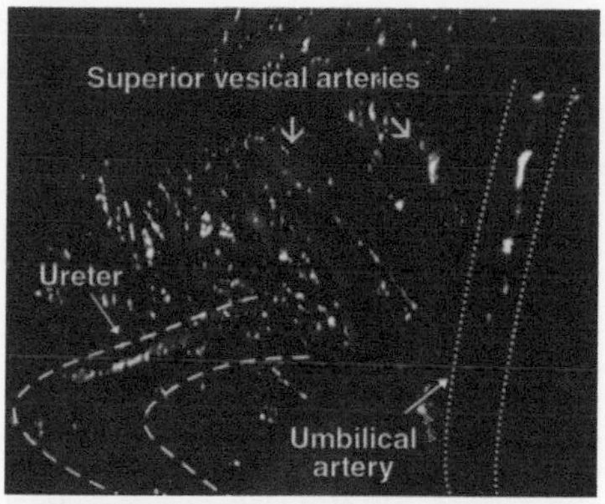

Figure 19.10 At this time, with a careful dissection, the superior vesical artery is found and isolated.

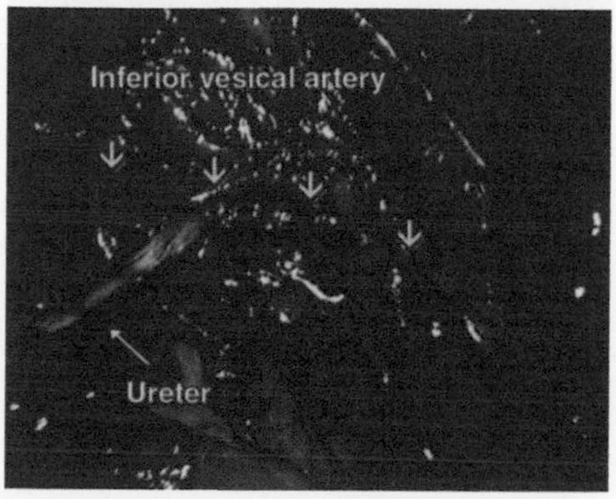

Figure 19.11 The inferior vesical artery can also be found and carefully dissected and isolated.

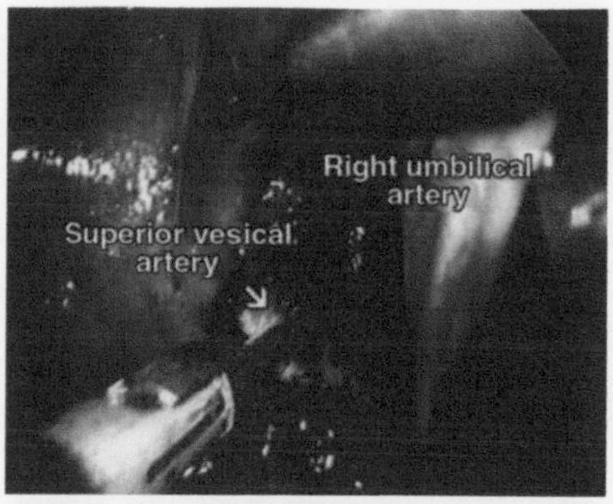

Figure 19.12 Both vesical arteries (superior and inferior) are controlled by the harmonic scalpel.

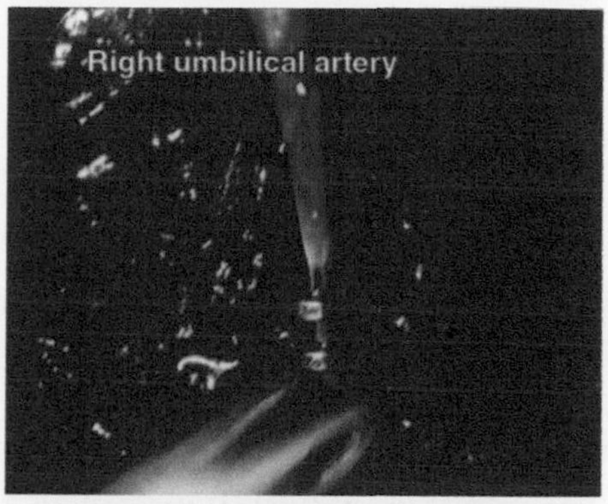

Figure 19.13 The right umbilical artery is clipped and transected at the origin from the deep iliac artery.

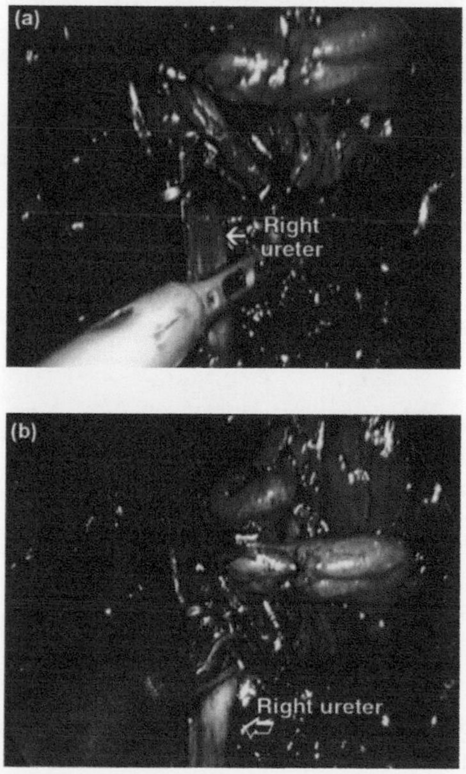

Figure 19.14 The right ureter is isolated as distally as possible, clamped between surgical clips, and cut, and the distal margin is send for frozen evaluation.

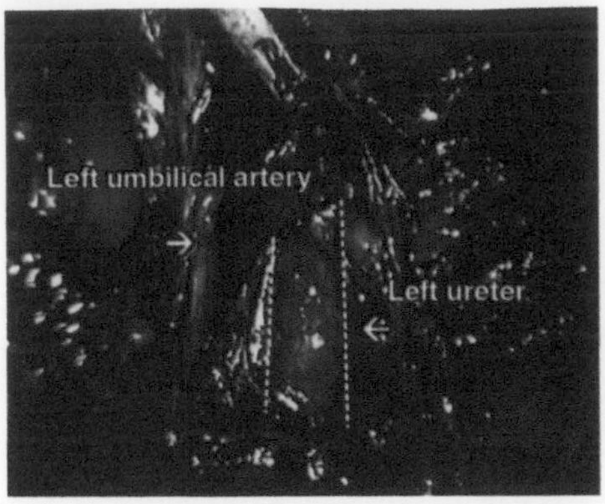

Figure 19.15 The same maneuver as in Figure 19.14 for the right side is carried out on the left side.

Endopelvic fascia incision and dorsal vein complex control

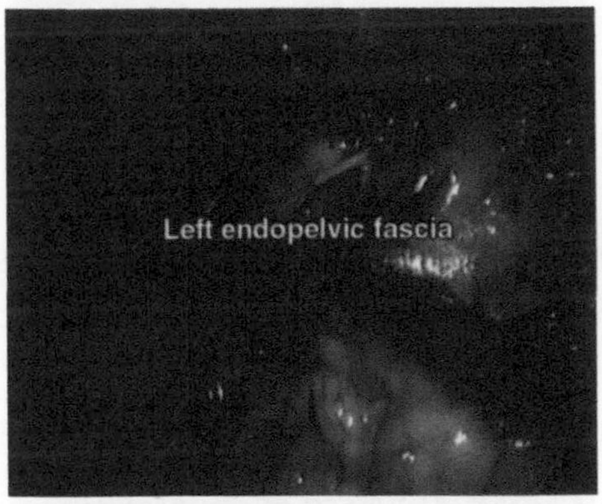

Figure 19.16 The anterior peritoneum is incised laterally to the umbilical arteries up to their junction with the urachus and the prevesical space is prepared dissecting the bladder from the anterior abdominal wall. The space is developed with sharp and blunt dissection until the endopelvic fascia is reached, and it is incised.

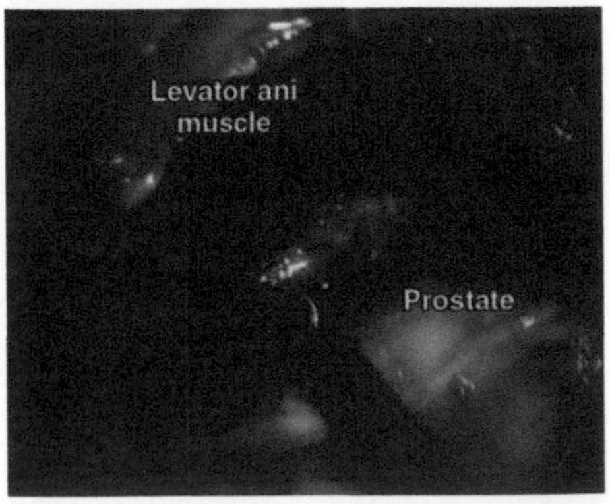

Figure 19.17 The incision is carried out on its reflection and the lateral surface of the prostate is dissected from the levator ani muscle to expose the lateral surface of the dorsal vein complex, the prostatic apex, and the urethra. A zero absorbable stitch is passed and the dorsal vein complex is secured.

Section of vesical and prostratic pedicles

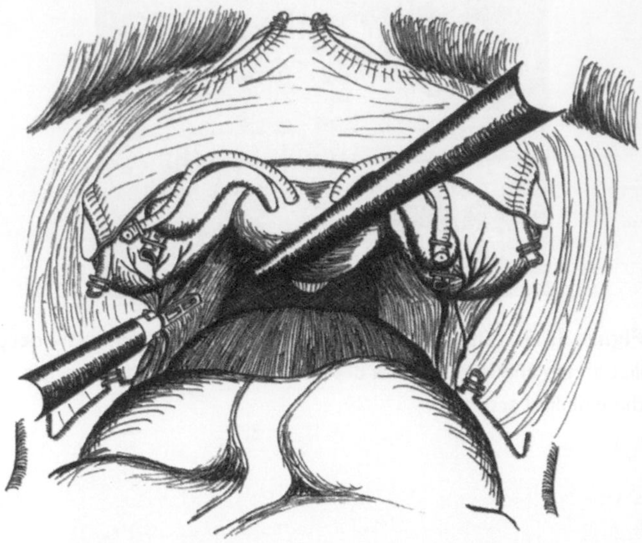

Figure 19.18 The suction device pulls up the vesico-prostatic complex, and the exposed vesico-prostatic pedicles are divided by harmonic scalpel. The pedicles appear like two tracks converging to the urethra; at the base of this tunnel lies the rectum.

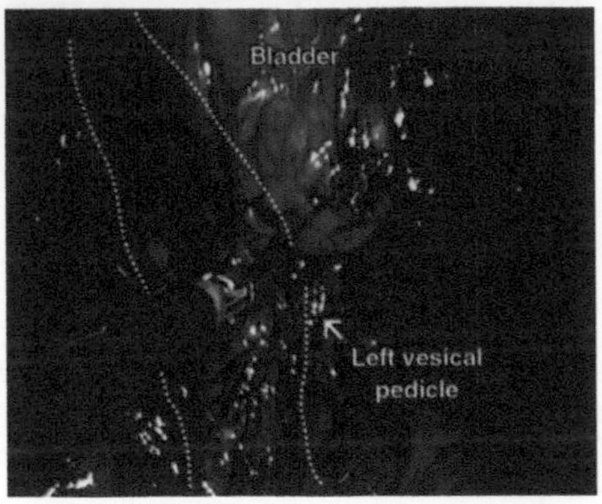

Figure 19.19 The first assistant pulls up the bladder with a grasper on the left hand while pushing the rectum down with the suction device to expose the left vesical pedicle. The pedicle is coagulated and divided with the harmonic scalpel.

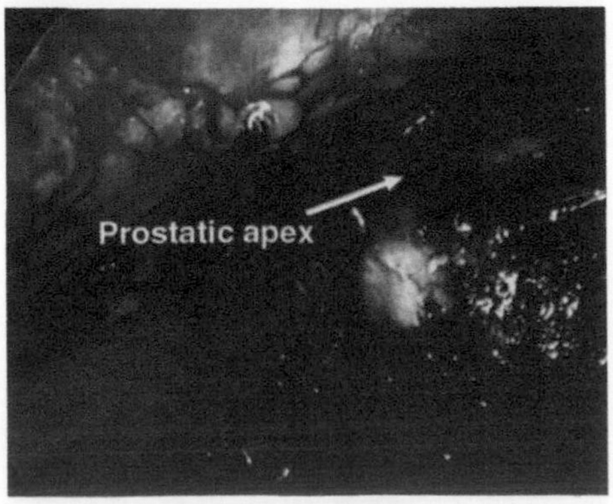

Figure 19.20 The dissection continues with the section of the prostatic pedicle and stops just proximally to the urethral sphincter.

Urethral section

At this point only the deep dorsal vein complex and the urethra fix the vesico-prostatic complex to the pelvic floor.

The incision is done as close as possible to the prostatic apex in order to have an adequate urethral stump.

After the external ligation of the distal end of the catheter, this is pulled into the abdominal cavity. The balloon is kept inflated to avoid urinary spillage, and the posterior wall of the urethra is cut.

The incision of the distal insertion of the Denonvillier's fascia completes the operation.

The specimen is inserted into an endoscopic bag.

Lymphadenectomy and specimen extraction

After lymphodenectomy the lymph nodes are entrapped inside a new endoscopic bag.

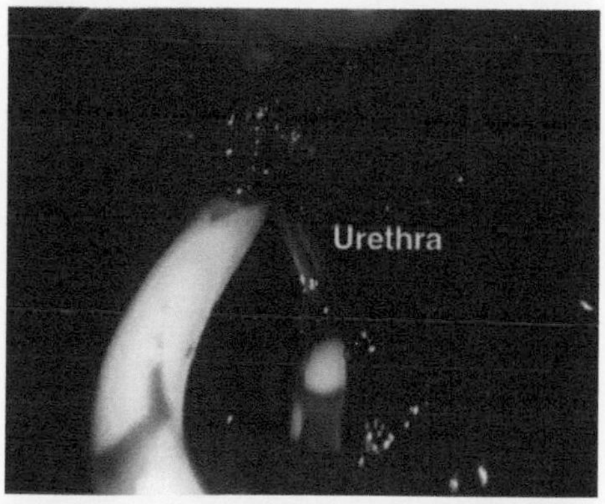

Figure 19.21 The dorsal vein complex is divided and the anterior urethral wall is incised.

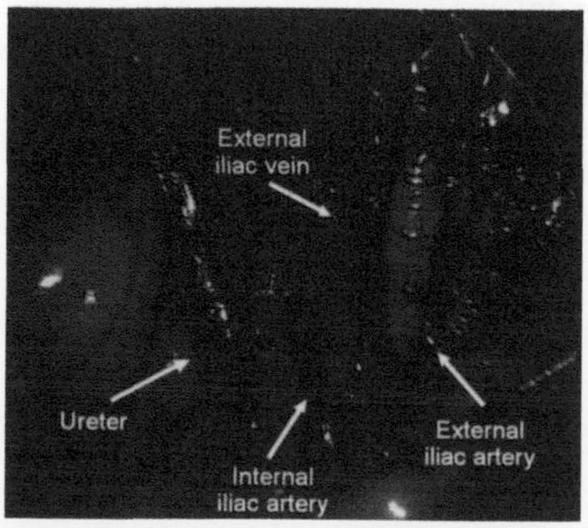

Figure 19.22 A bilateral extended pelvic lymphadenectomy is then performed. The boundaries are: laterally the external iliac artery and genito-femoral nerve, distally the inguinal ligament, medially the hypogastric artery, and proximally the bifurcation of the common iliac arteries.

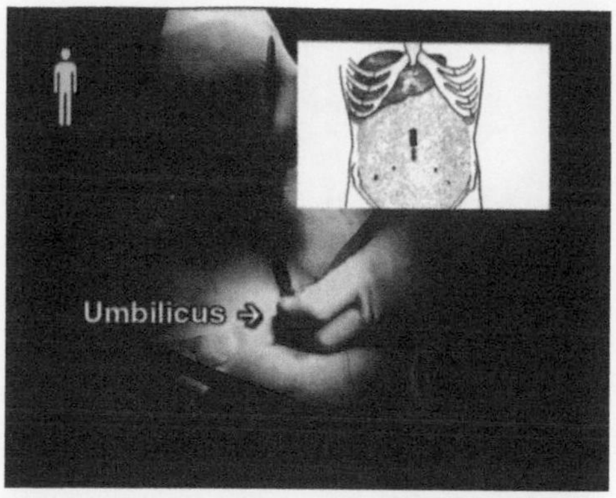

Figure 19.23 In case of a planned ileal neobladder, a supra-umbilical incision of 5 cm is carried out to extract both bags. The five trocars are left in place so that the urinary diversion can be performed later.

Urinary diversion

Different urinary diversions have been described in the literature, i.e., uretero-cutaneostomy,[1,9] Bricker,[2,10] Mainz II,[3,7] or different types of ileal neobladder – Studer,[4,10] MILaN,[5] performed partially[5,6] or completely intracorporeally.[4,10] We describe a technique of ileal neobladder partially performed extracorporeally, known as MILaN.[5]

It is possible to perform the neobladder reconstruction and the uretero–neobladder anastomosis completely extracorporeally. In this case, it is better to perform the skin abdominal incision in an inferior position with respect to the umbilicus, only the urethral–neobladder anastomosis is performed intracorporeally.

If only the partially fashioned neobladder is reinserted with the intestinal anastomosis into the abdominal cavity, the supra-umbilical incision is sutured and the pneumoperitoneum is created in order to continue and complete the neobladder reconstruction.

POSTOPERATIVE SCHEDULE

The operative time is about 100–150 minutes for the cystectomy and 30–250 minutes for the diversion (shortest for ureterocutaneostomy, longest for ileal neobladder).

The blood loss is reduced with respect to the open technique and the postoperative pain is negligible.

Bowel activity is rapid, usually postoperative day 2–3, and food intake is usually 2 days later. The drain is removed early (2–4 days postoperatively).

In case of ileal neobladder, the single J indwelling catheter is removed after radiographic assessment on day 7–10. The catheter in the neobladder is usually removed 7 days later.

The only unresolved problem is the oncological follow-up. At present this is not long enough to permit a conclusion to be drawn as to whether this procedure can be considered a real alternative to the open technique.

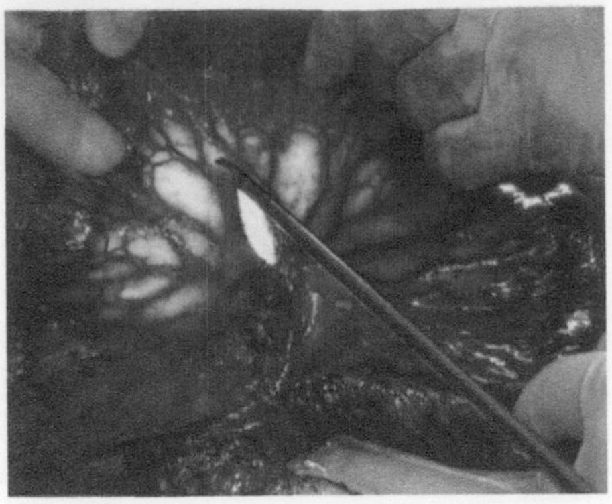

Figure 19.24 The ileum is extracted through the 5 cm supra-umbilical abdominal incision and 25 cm of it is isolated 15 cm proximal to the ileocecal junction. The harmonic scalpel is used to close the arteries and veins using standard transillumination technique.

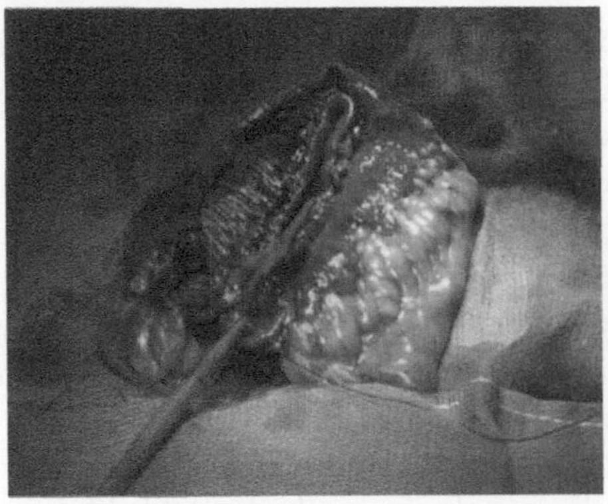

Figure 19.25 External stapled side-to-side anastomosis is performed with external reapproximation of the mesenteric margins to avoid ileus due to an internal hernia. The external isolated ileal segment is detubularized, cleaned, and partially fashioned.

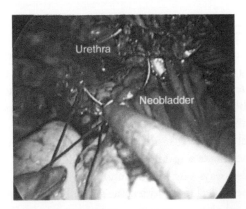

Figure 19.26 The neobladder is anastomos with the urethra with six to eight single 2/0 absorbable stitches; a Beniquet sound can help during the creation of the anastomosis, for better visualization and creation of a water-tight reapproximation. The fixation of the neobladder to the urethra is helpful for carrying out the subsequent uretero–neobladder anastomosis.

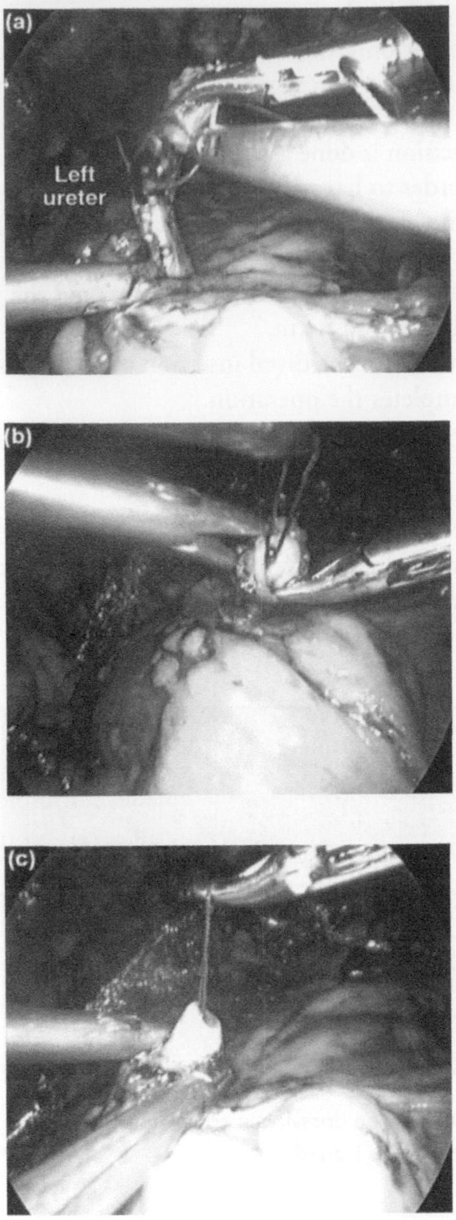

Figure 19.27 If the ureter is normal a direct anastomosis can be done. In case of a dilated ureter a non-refluxing anastomosis is created using a nipple mechanism as described by Simonata et al.[11] After the insertion of a guidewire, two single J stents are inserted into the ureters to protect the anastomoses.

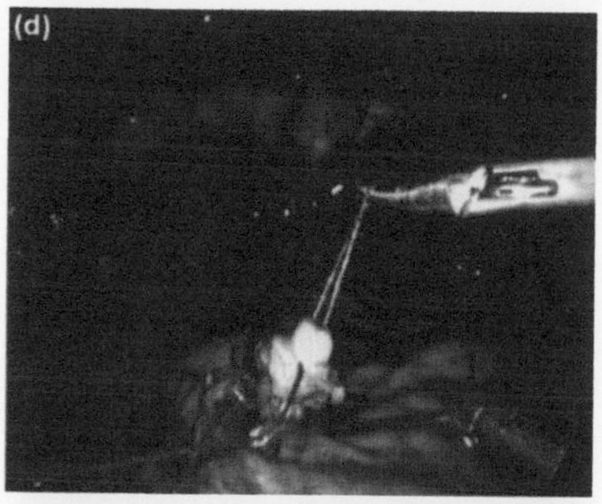

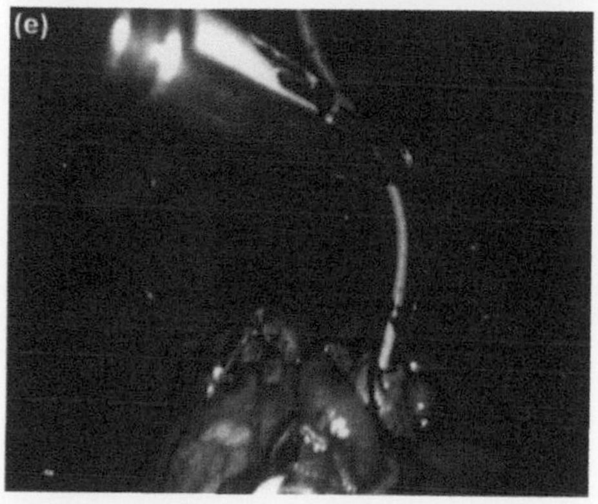

Figure 19.27 Continued.

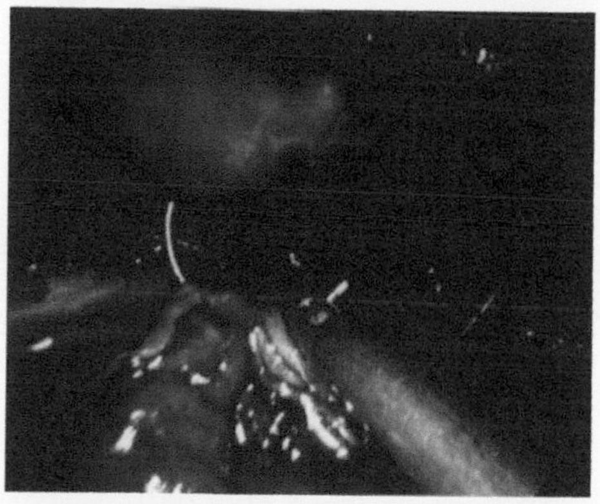

Figure 19.28 A 20Fr Foley catheter is inserted and the anterior wall of the neobladder is closed with a 2/0 absorbable running suture. The bladder is filled with 100–150 ml of saline to check the water-tightness of the sutures, and a pelvic drain is placed.

REFERENCES

1. Puppo P, Perachino M, Ricciotti G et al. Laparoscopically assisted transvaginal radical cystectomy. Eur Urol 1995; 27: 80–4.
2. Gill I, Fergany A, Klein E et al. Laparoscopic radical cystoprostatectomy with ileal conduit performed completely intracorporeally: the initial 2 cases. Urology 2000; 56: 26–9.
3. Tuerk I, Deger S, Winkelmann B et al. Laparoscopic radical cystectomy with continent urinary diversion (rectal sigmoid pouch) performed completely intracorporeally. The initial 5 cases. J Urol 2001; 165: 1863–6.
4. Gill I, Kaouk J, Meraney A et al. Laparoscopic radical cystectomy and continent orthotopic ileal neobladder performed completely intracorporeally: the initial experience. J Urol 2002; 168: 13–18.
5. Gaboardi F, Simonato A, Galli S et al. Minimally invasive laparoscopic neobladder. J Urol 2002; 168: 1080–3.
6. Adbel-hakim AM, Bassiouny F, Azim M et al. Laparoscopic radical cystectomy with orthotopic neobladder. J Endourol 2002; 16: 377–81.
7. Deger S, Peters R, Roigas J, Loening S. Laparoscopic radical cystectomy with continent urinary diversion (recto-sigmoid pouch) performed completely intracorporeally: an intermediate functional and oncologic analysis. Urology 2004; 64: 935–9.
8. Simonato A, Gregori A, Lissiani A et al. Laparoscopic radical cystectomy: a technique illustrated step by step. Eur Urol 2003; 44: 132–8.
9. Simonato A, Gregori A, Lissiani A et al. Laparoscopic radical cystoprostatectomy: our experience in a consecutive series of 10 patients with 3 years follow-up. Eur Urol 2005; 47: 785–92.
10. Haber G, Colombo J, Aron M et al. Laparoscopic radical cystectomy and urinary diversion: status 2006. Eur Urol 2006; Suppl 19: 950–5.
11. Simonato A, Gregori A, Lissiani A et al. Intracorporeal uretero-enteric anastomosis during laparoscopic continent urinary diversion. BJU Int 2004; 93: 1351–4.

CHAPTER 20

Radical cystectomy in the female patient

Franco Gaboardi, Ioannis Goumas-Kartalas, Stefano Galli, and Andrea Gregori

The treatment of choice for muscle invasive bladder cancer is radical cystectomy.[1] In the female, anterior pelvic exenteration with en bloc removal of the bladder, uterus, fallopian tubes, ovaries, and anterior vaginal wall represented the standard technique for many years. In the last decade it has been proved that a less destructive procedure with orthotopic neobladder reconstruction is oncologically safe in selected cases.[2] Laparoscopic radical cystectomy in the female has been reported in the literature[3,4] and we know now that it is technically feasible, with a promising short-term oncologic follow-up. We propose a step-by-step description of the technique of laparoscopic radical cystectomy in the female. The procedure can be divided as follows:

1. Patient preparation
2. Laparoscopic access
3. Laparoscopic radical cystectomy
   a) Laparoscopic extended anterior pelvic exenteration
   b) Nerve-sparing radical cystectomy with preservation of the vagina or uterus and conservation of the urethra for orthotopic neobladder reconstruction
4. Pelvic lymphadenectomy
5. Urinary diversion.

PATIENT PREPARATION

As in the male patient, the bowel is prepared by oral administration of 2 litres of electrolyte lavage. Antibiotic prophylaxis and low-molecular-weight heparin are administered preoperatively.

The patient is placed in the supine position with the legs apart and the table is set in moderate Trendelenburg position. The surgeon is on the left side of the table with the first assistant in front and the second assistant (for the laparoscope) on the right of the first assistant. The nurse is on the left of the surgeon. The anesthetist is at the patient's head.

LAPAROSCOPIC ACCESS

Similar to the male patient, a five port fan-shaped transperitoneal access is used. The first 12 mm trocar, reserved for the laparoscope, is placed with an open technique through a mini-laparotomy on the right side of the umbilicus. The remaining four ports (one 12 mm and three 5 mm) are placed under endoscopic control after establishment of the pneumoperitoneum. The abdomen and the pelvis are carefully inspected.

LAPAROSCOPIC EXTENDED ANTERIOR PELVIC EXENTERATION WITHOUT PRESERVATION OF THE URETHRA AND ANTERIOR WALL OF THE VAGINA

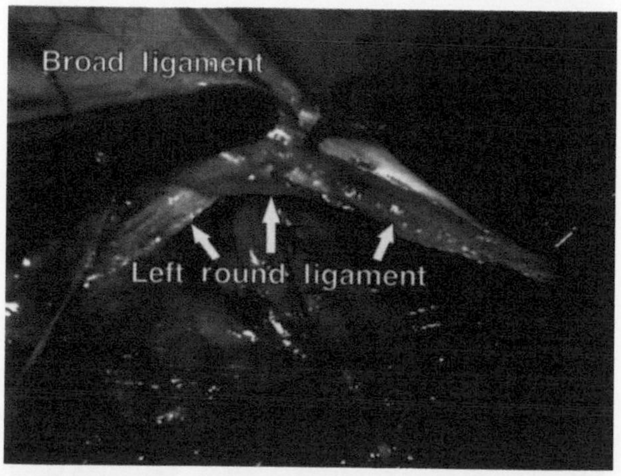

Figure 20.1 After incision of the broad ligament, the round ligament is isolated and transected.

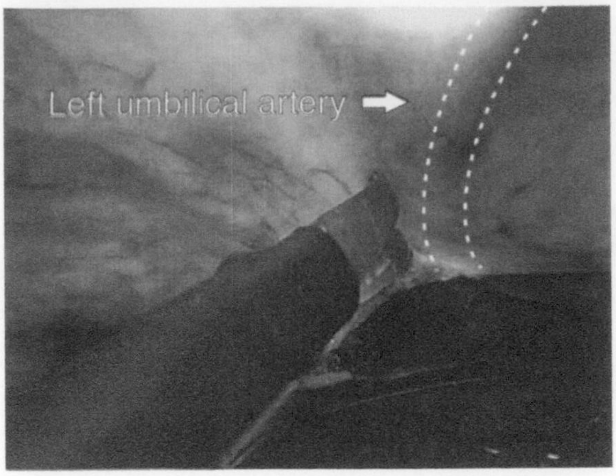

Figure 20.2 The anterior peritoneum is opened just laterally to the left umbilical artery.

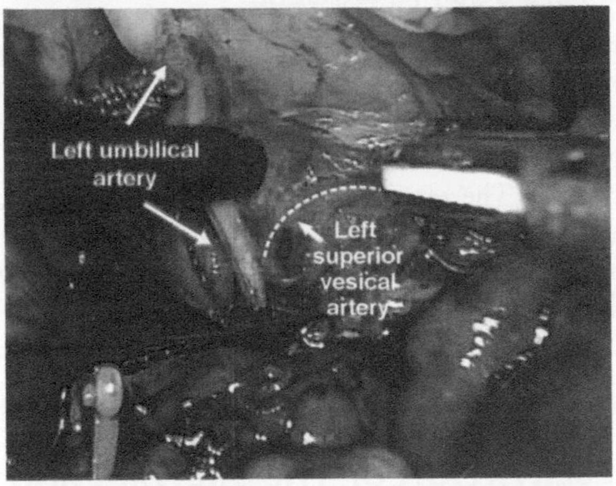

Figure 20.3 The dissection proceeds in a retrograde fashion following the left umbilical artery. In this way, the first branch of the internal iliac artery, the superior vesical artery, can be easily identified and transected.

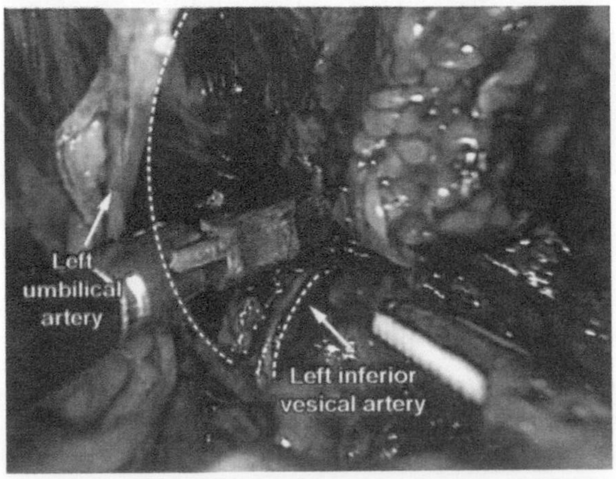

Figure 20.4 The inferior vesical artery is identified and controlled with the harmonic scalpel.

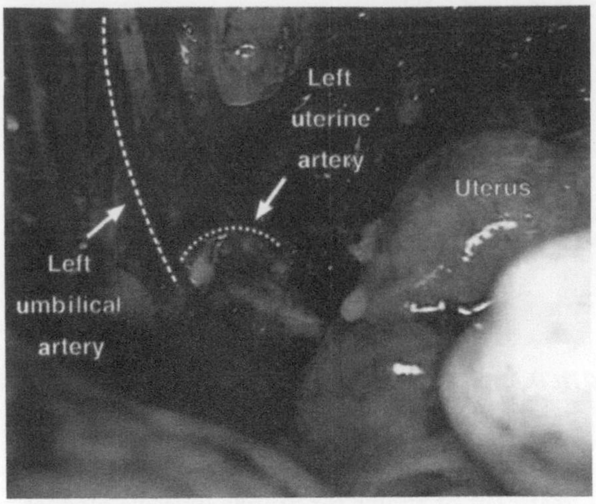

Figure 20.5 Proximally, the uterine artery is identified, clamped, and transected.

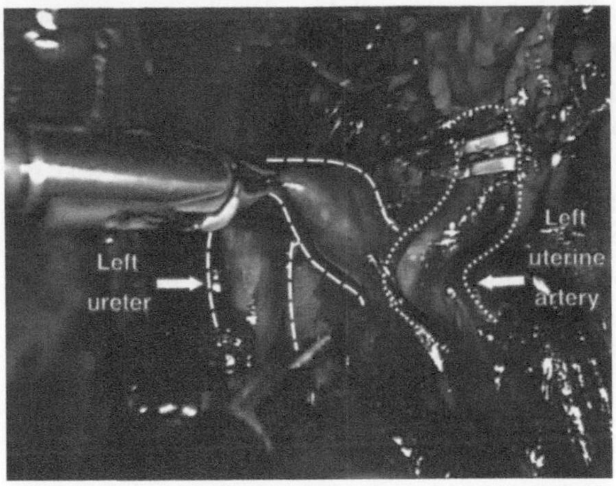

Figure 20.6 After dividing the uterine artery, the ureter can be identified.

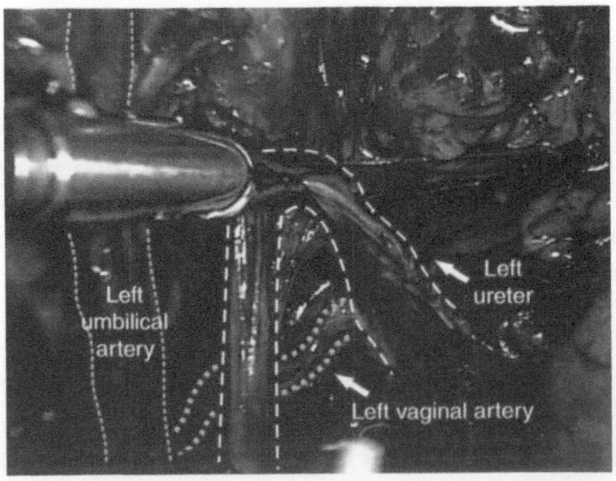

Figure 20.7 The dissection is then carried down to the pelvic ureter near the terminal branches of the uterine artery. At this level the vaginal artery can be identified and controlled.

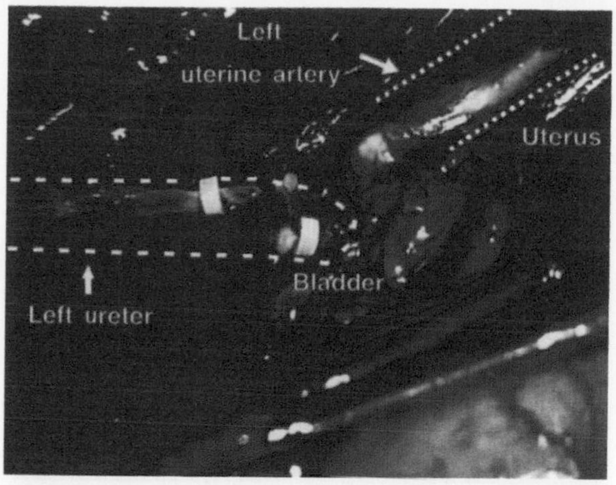

Figure 20.8 The ureter is isolated until its insertion to the bladder. After clamping with Hem-o-Loks, the ureter is divided and the distal margin is sent for frozen section evaluation. The same procedure is then performed on the left side.

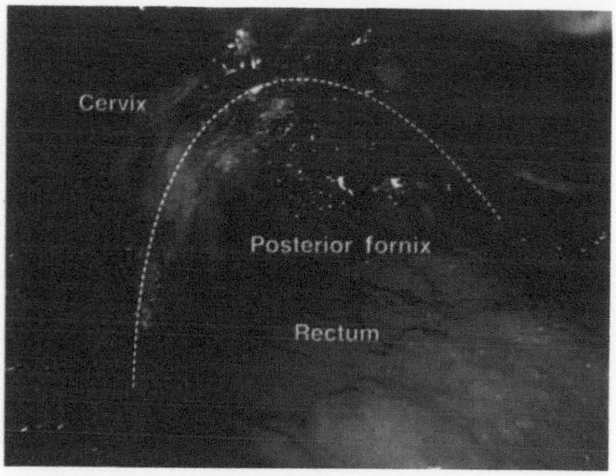

Figure 20.11 The posterior vaginal wall can be mobilized off the rectum with the aid of a simple metallic retractor within the vagina.

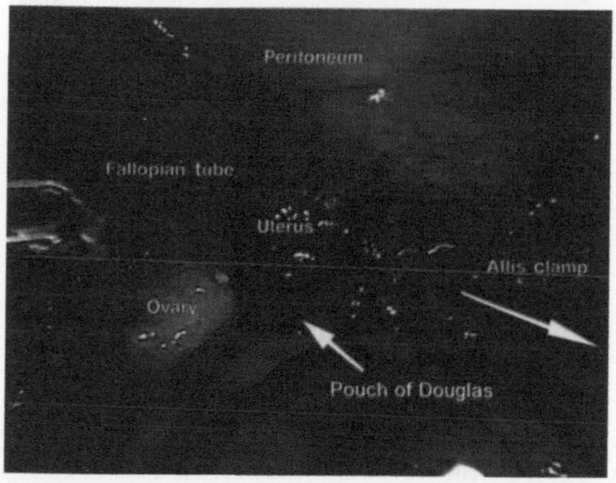

Figure 20.9 The uterus is retracted cranially with an Allis clamp and the pouch of Douglas is identified.

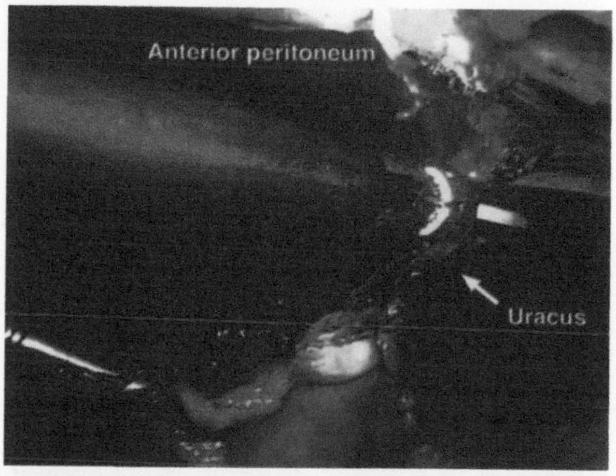

Figure 20.12 The incision of the anterior peritoneum is performed laterally to the umbilical arteries on both sides. The urachus is incised.

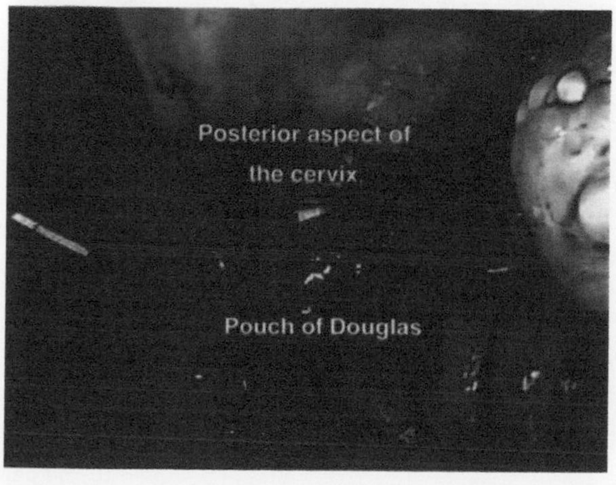

Figure 20.10 Incision of the utero-sacral ligaments is carried out bilaterally and a good exposure of the cul de sac is obtained.

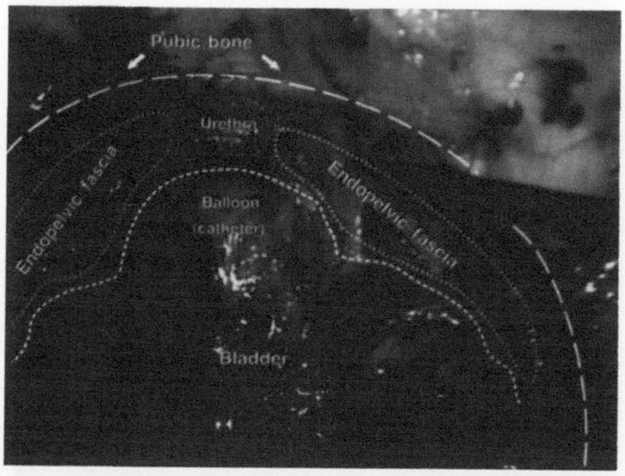

Figure 20.13 The Retzius space is opened and the bladder is mobilized to obtain a good exposure of the endopelvic fascia, which is subsequently open on both sides of the bladder.

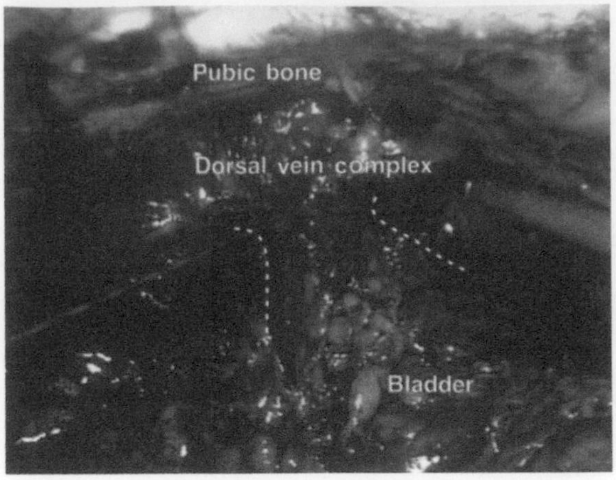

Figure 20.14 The dorsal vein complex of the clitoris is identified and ligated with a 0 polyglactin stitch using a CT-1 needle.

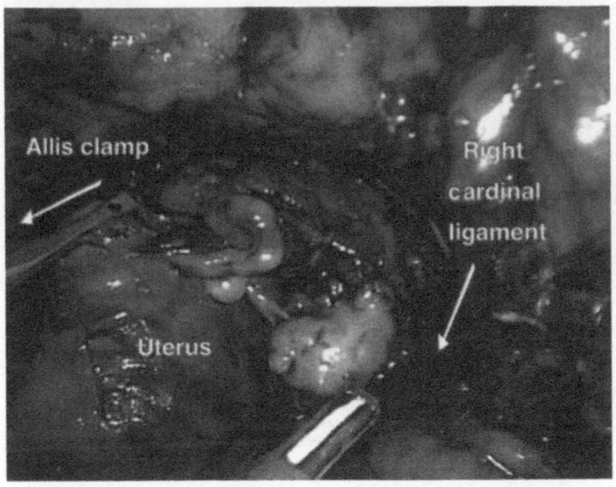

Figure 20.15 The uterus can be mobilized laterally and cranially using an Allis clamp to expose the cardinal ligaments.

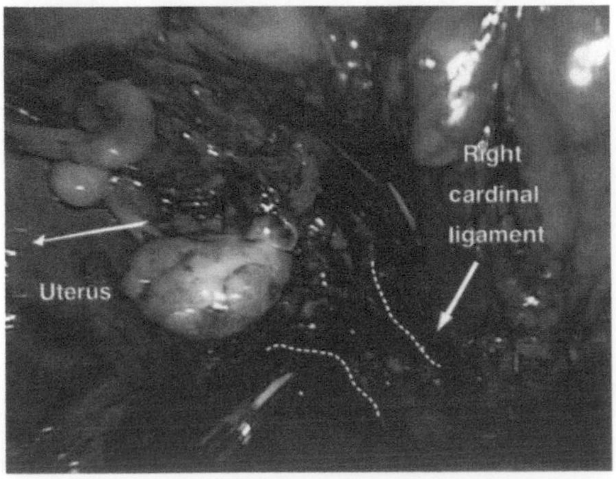

Figure 20.16 The cardinal ligaments are isolated.

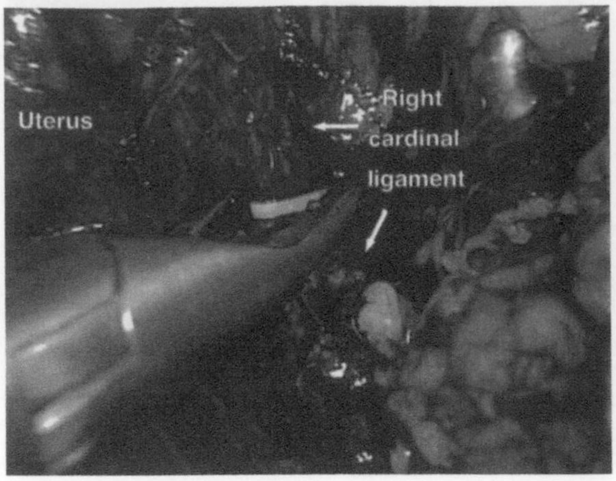

Figure 20.17 The cardinal ligaments are clipped with Hem-o-Loks and transected with the harmonic scalpel.

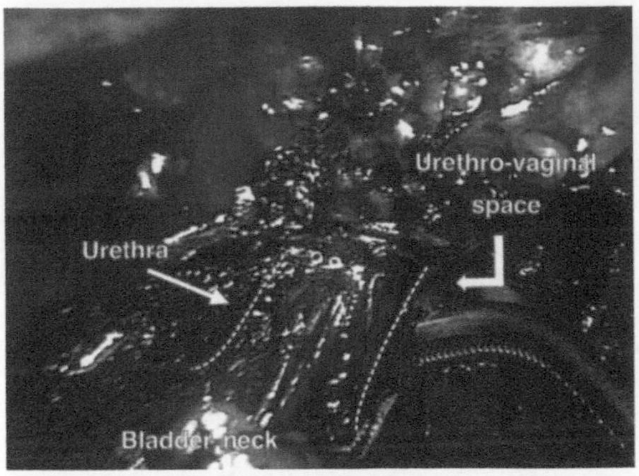

Figure 20.18 The urethra is isolated and the the urethro-vaginal space is prepared using a right angle.

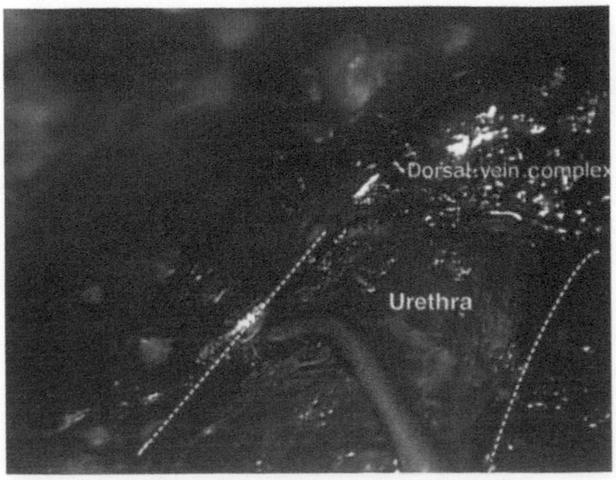

Figure 20.19 The urethra is clamped and divided as distally as possible.

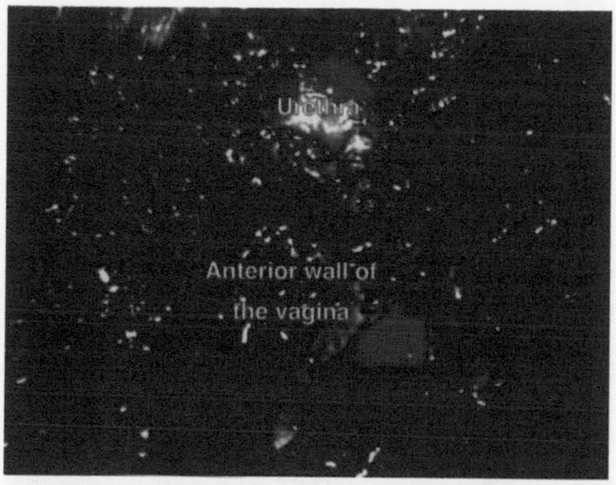

Figure 20.20 After dividing the urethra, the anterior vaginal wall is exposed.

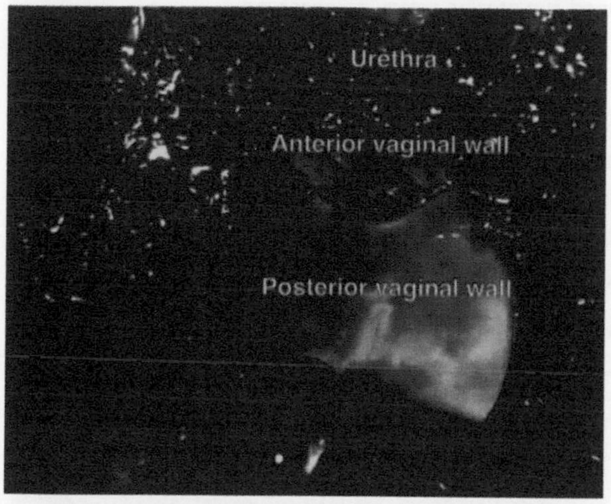

Figure 20.21 The anterior vaginal wall is transected transversally until the lateral vaginal walls are reached.

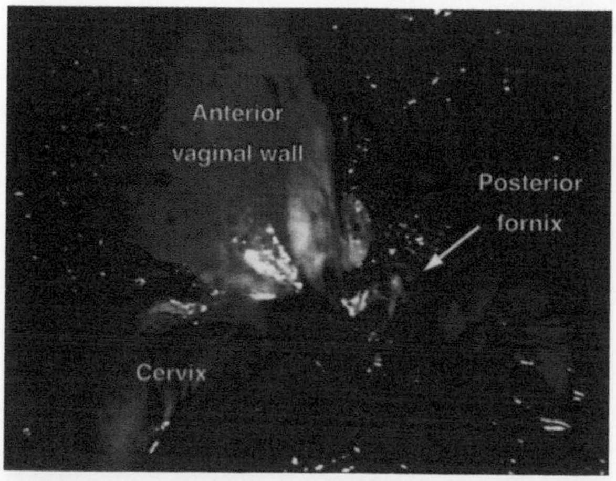

Figure 20.22 The dissection proceeds cranially towards the anterior fornix. At this level, the incision continues vertically towards the posterior fornix. The entire excision of the anterior vaginal wall is completed after transection of the posterior fornix.

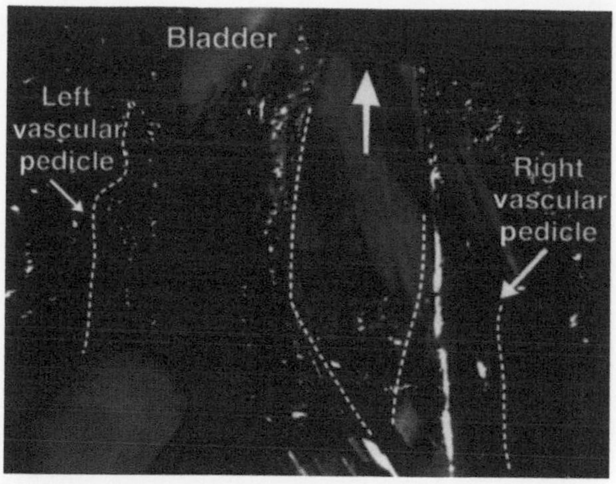

Figure 20.23 The bladder is easily moved cranially. This maneuver helps in identifying the vascular pedicles.

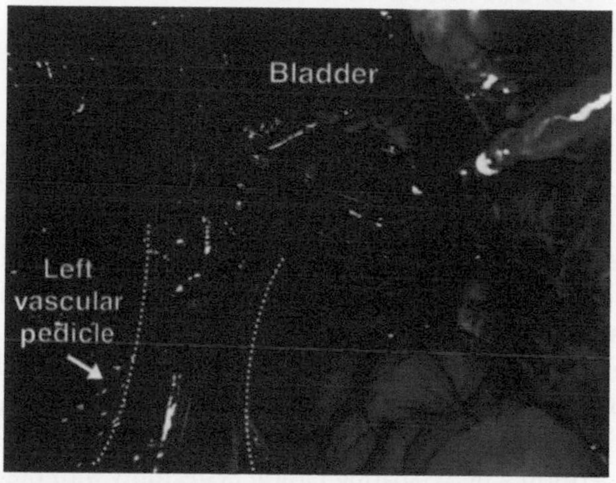

Figure 20.24 The vascular pedicles are transected with the harmonic scalpel. The en bloc cystohysteroannessiectomy is perfomed.

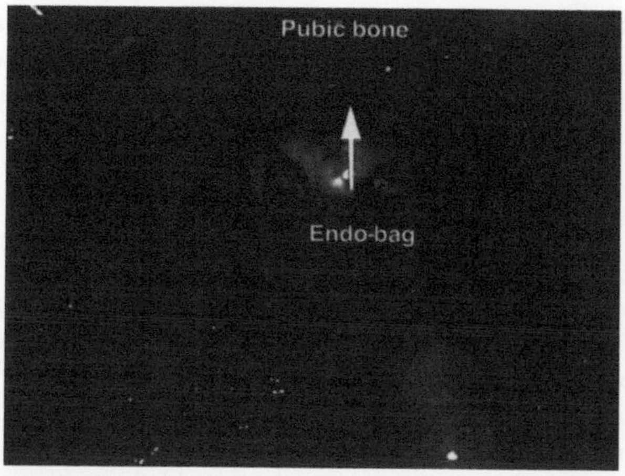

Figure 20.25 An endo-bag is introduced into the abdominal cavity through the opened vagina and the surgical specimen is removed.

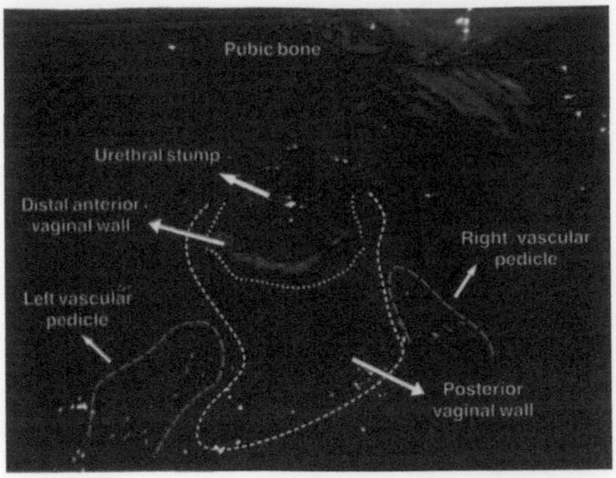

Figure 20.26 At the end of the anterior exenteration the posterior and part of the lateral vaginal walls can be seen.

NERVE-SPARING RADICAL CYSTECTOMY WITH URETHRA PRESERVATION (UTERUS OR VAGINA SPARING)

The available literature supports the performance of an orthotopic urinary diversion in appropriately selected women following radical cystectomy for primary bladder malignancy.[2,5] From an oncologic point of view, preoperative absence of tumor in the bladder neck and vagina and a negative full-thickness intraoperative frozen section analysis of the proximal urethra indicate the preservation of the urethra with neobladder reconstruction.[6] The detailed topographic anatomy of the pelvic autonomic nerves innervating the vagina, urethra, and bladder allows the surgeon to perform a nerve-sparing radical cystectomy with preservation of the vagina and in some selected cases of the uterus, in order to preserve sexual function in females.[2,5,7,8]

PELVIC LYMPHADENECTOMY

Extended pelvic lymphadenectomy is performed according to the standard procedure at the end of radical cystectomy, as described in Chapter 19 for the procedure in the male.[9,10]

URINARY DIVERSION

After extended anterior exenteration, the specimen can be removed throughout the open vagina. Various options for urinary diversions include cutaneous ureterostomy, sigmoid ureterostomy (Mainz II), or ileal conduit.[11–13] Urinary diversion can be performed extracorporeally or intracorporeally.

In case of preservation of urethra, neobladder orthotopic reconstruction is performed either extracorporeally or intracorporeally. Our technique (MILaN) has been described previously.[14] Although other authors have described a

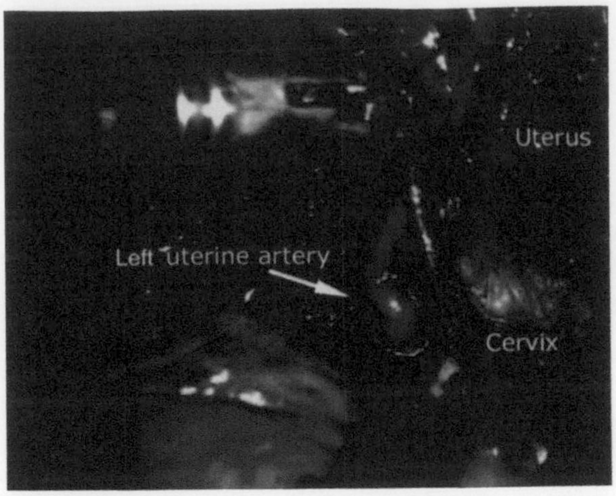

Figure 20.27 The bladder is mobilized off the uterus using the harmonic scalpel. Dissection is easily conducted between the uterine artery and the distal ureter. If a uterus-sparing procedure is planned, the uterine artery is conserved.

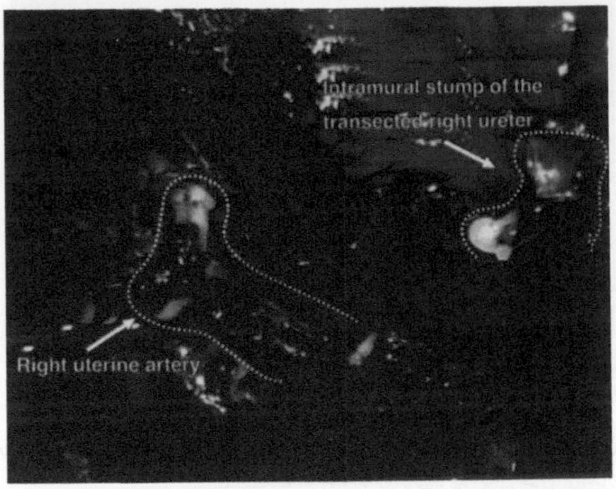

Figure 20.28 If a hysterectomy is planned, the uterine artery is clipped and transected, followed by the transection of the ureter (the right uterine artery and ureter can be seen).

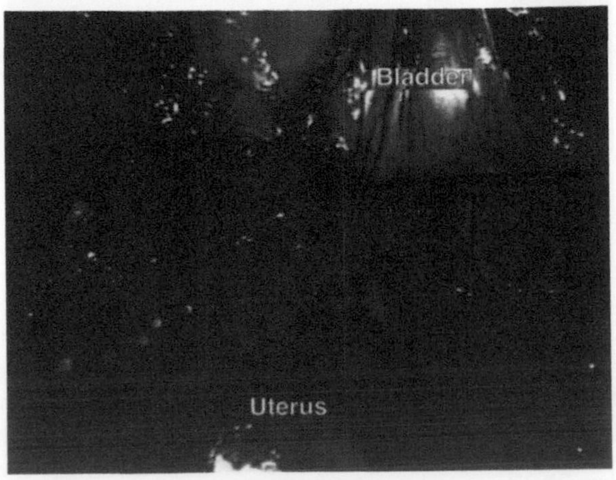

Figure 20.29 The utero-vesical space is entered.

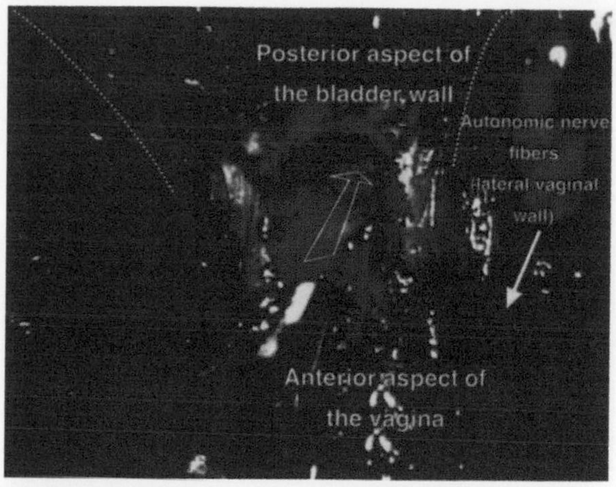

Figure 20.30 Dissection of the vesico-vaginal space proceeds until the level of the bladder wall. Caution must be made to avoid damaging the autonomic nerve fibers located at the lateral vaginal walls.

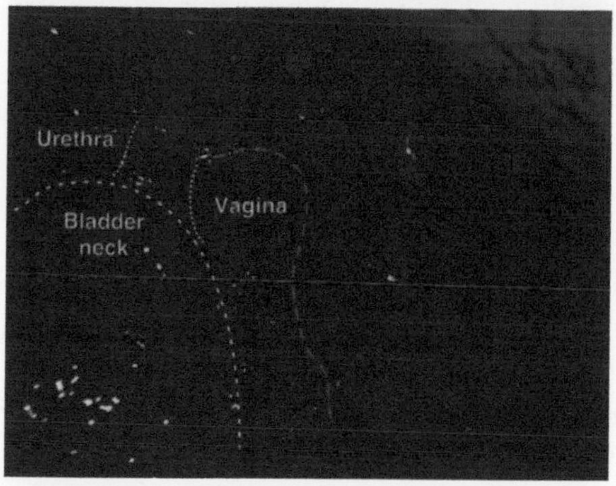

Figure 20.31 At this point, the urethra can be clearly identified.

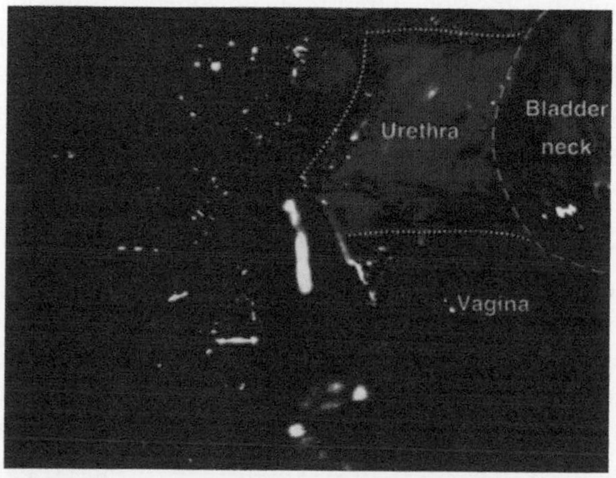

Figure 20.32 Isolation of the urethra is performed with caution in order to avoid damage to the rhabdomyosphincter.

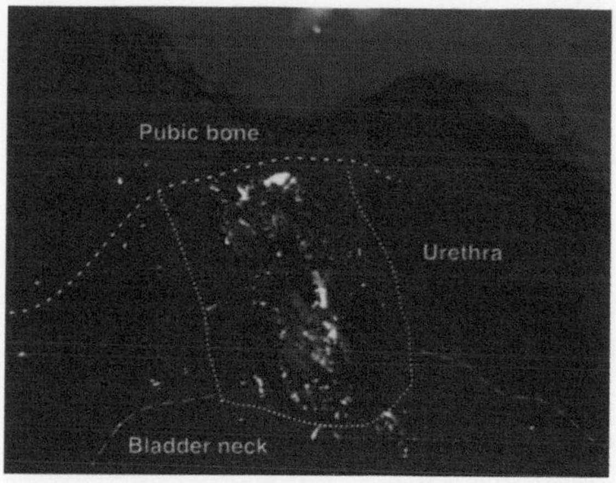

Figure 20.33 The anterior wall of the urethra is incised at about 1 cm below the bladder neck, leaving the caudal portion of the urethra and the rhabdomyosphincter intact.

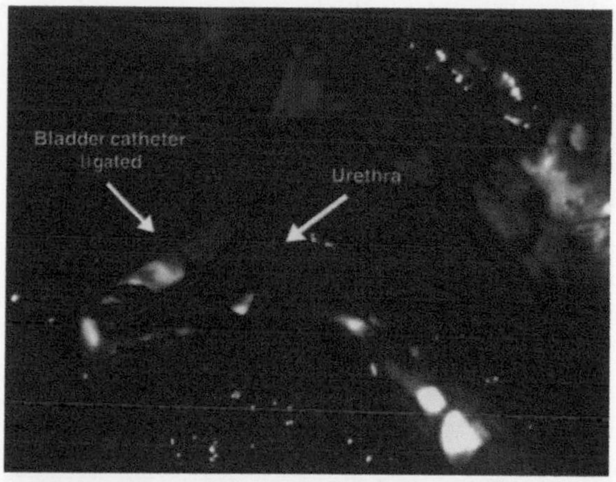

Figure 20.34 After incision of the anterior wall of the urethra, the catheter, previously cut and clamped from the outside to avoid any urine spillage, is exposed and pulled into the abdominal cavity. With a gentle traction on the catheter the posterior wall of the urethra is sectioned and cystectomy is completed. The endo-bag with the bladder alone is removed through the abdominal wall.

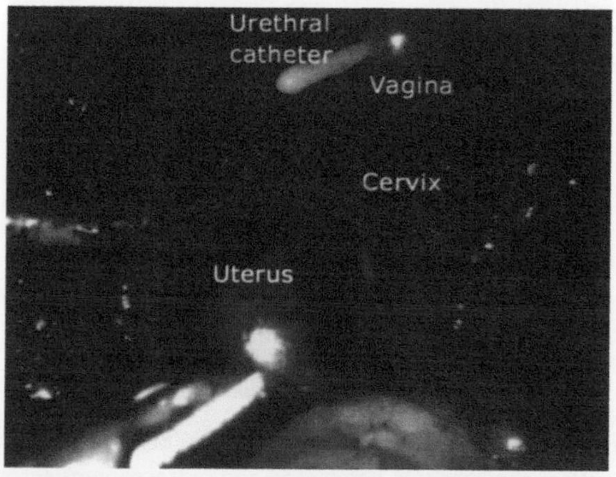

Figure 20.35 After removing the bladder alone through the abdominal wall, we can identify the uterus and vagina, which have been spared (uterus-sparing cystectomy).

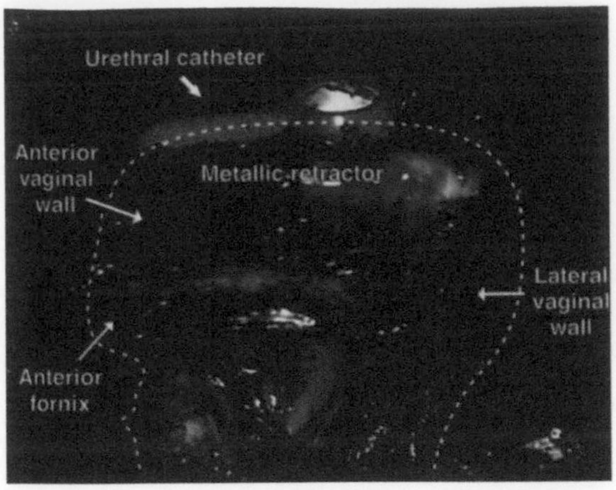

Figure 20.36 When a hysteroannesiectomy is planned with conservation of the vagina, we proceed with a nerve-sparing vaginal dissection. A small catheter is then placed in the urethra and the balloon is inflated with 5 ml to maintain the pneumoperitoneum. A gentle traction with a malleable retractor is provided so as to locate and section the anterior fornix of the vagina.

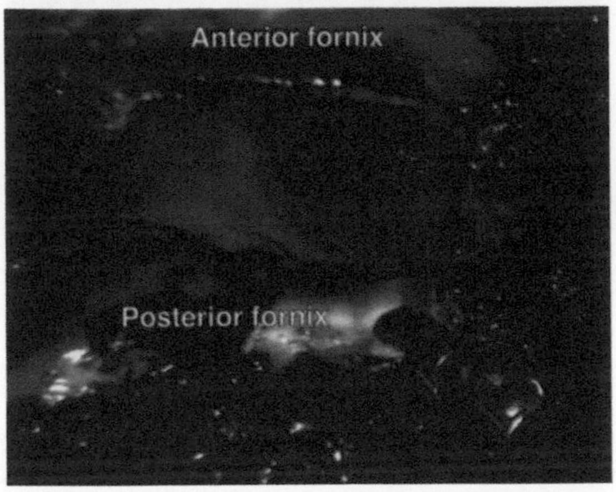

Figure 20.37 The incision proceeds circumferentially towards the posterior fornix.

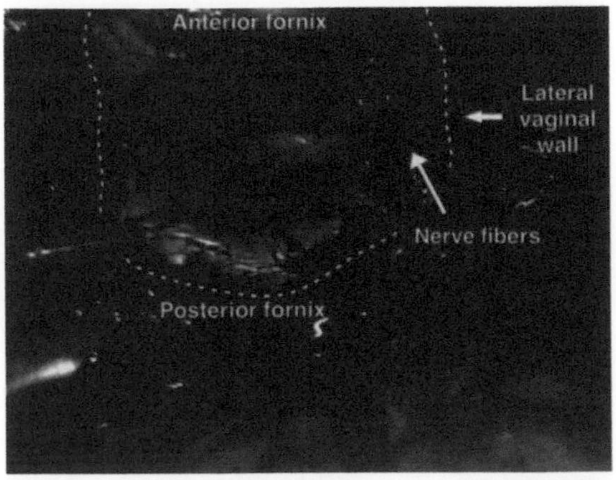

Figure 20.38 The circumferential incision of the vaginal wall at the level of the fornix is completed and hysteroannessiectomy is performed. The vagina and the autonomic nerve fibers located at the lateral vaginal walls remain intact (nerve-sparing radical cystectomy with vagina conservation).

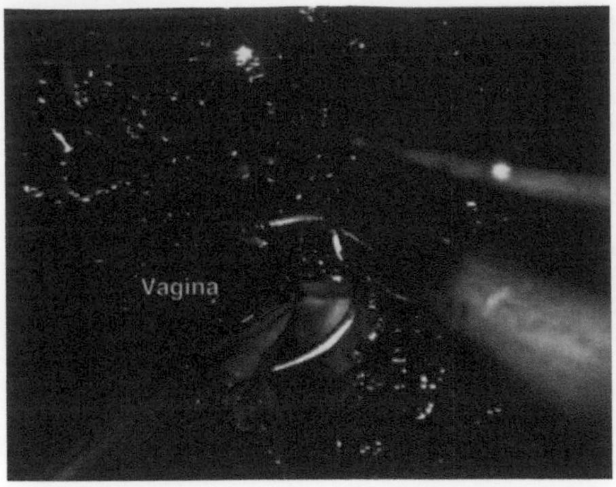

Figure 20.39 Reconstruction of the vagina in a transverse way begins with a 2/0 vicryl running suture.

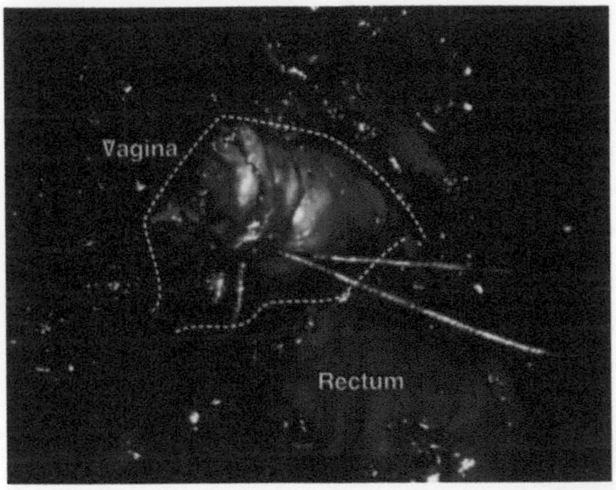

Figure 20.40 Final aspect of the reconstructed vagina for preservation of sexual function.

totally intracorporeal neobladder reconstruction,[15] we prefer a combined extracorporeal and intracorporeal technique, with exteriorization of the bowel through a small abdominal incision. Urethro–neobladder anastomosis is performed laparoscopically. In our opinion with this technique the operative time is reduced and the operative field remains clear of bowel secretions during the neobladder reconstruction.

POSTOPERATIVE SCHEDULE

The operative time for laparoscopic radical cystectomy in female patients, blood loss, time to oral intake, and hospital stay are similar to the results of laparoscopic radical cystectomy in male patients. The overall cases of laparoscopic radical cystectomy in female patients are fewer than those in male patients. A longer follow-up is required in order to evaluate accurately the functional outcomes and oncologic results.

REFERENCES

1. Stein JP, Lieskovsky G, Cote R et al. Radical cystectomy in the treatment of invasive bladder cancer: long-term results in 1,054 patients. J Clin Oncol 2001; 19(3): 666–75.
2. Stenzl A, Colleselli K, Poisel S et al. Rationale and technique of nerve-sparing radical cystectomy before an orthotopic neobladder procedure in women. J Urol 1995; 154: 2044–9.
3. Moinzadeh A, Gill IS, Desai M et al. Laparoscopic radical cystectomy in the female. J Urol 2005; 173: 1912–17.
4. Menon M, Hemal AK, Shrivastava A et al. Robot-assisted radical cystectomy and urinary diversion in female patients: technique with preservation of the uterus and vagina. J Am Coll Surg 2004; 198(3): 386–93.
5. Nagele U, Kuczyk M, Anastasiadis AG et al. Radical cystectomy and orthotopic bladder replacement in females. Eur Urol 2006; 50: 249–57.
6. Wu SD, Simma-Chang V, Stein JP. Pathologic guidelines for orthotopic urinary diversion in women with bladder cancer: a review of the literature. Rev Urol 2006; 8(2): 54–60.
7. Yukel S, De Souza A, Baskin LS. Neuroanatomy of the human female lower urogenital tract. J Urol 2004; 172: 191–5.
8. Yukel S, Baskin LS. An anatomical description of the male and female urethral sphincter complex. J Urol 2004; 171: 1890–7.
9. Herr H, Lee C, Chang S, Lerner S. Standardization of radical cystectomy and pelvic lymph node dissection for bladder cancer: a collaborative group report. J Urol 2004; 171: 1823–8.
10. Finelli A, Gill IS, Desai MM et al. Laparosocpic extended pelvic lymphadenectomy for bladder cancer: technique and initial outcomes. J Urol 2004; 172: 1809–12.
11. Puppo P, Perachino M, Ricciotti G et al. Laparoscopically assisted transvaginal radical cystectomy. Eur Urol 1995; 27: 80–4.
12. Deger S, Peters R, Roigas J, Loening S. Laparoscopic radical cystectomy with continent urinary diversion (recto-sigmoid pouch) performed completely intracorporeally: an intermediate functional and oncologic analysis. Urology 2004; 64: 935–9.
13. Gill I, Fergany A, Klein E et al. Laparoscopic radical cystoprostatectomy with ileal conduit performed completely intracorporeally: the initial 2 cases. Urology 2000; 56: 26–9.
14. Gaboardi F, Simonato A, Galli S et al. Minimally invasive laparoscopic neobladder. J Urol 2002; 168: 1080–3.
15. Gill IS, Kaouk JH, Meraney AM et al. Laparoscopic radical cystectomy and continent orthotopic ileal neobladder performed completely intracorporeally: the initial experience. J Urol 2002; 168: 13–8.

Index

Note: Page references in *italics* refer to Figures and Tables

Printed and bound by CPI Group (UK) Ltd, Croydon, CR0 4YY
23/10/2024
01777995-0001